MW01154808

Play Therapy Activities for Toddlers

101 Fun Games and Exercises to Enhance Motor Skills, Emotional Regulation, and Problem-Solving Abilities While Strengthening Your Bond

Table of Contents

Introduction

Have you ever been amazed by how dynamic your toddler is? One second, they're a bundle of laughs. The next, they're a storm of tears. There's so much potential within that tiny personality of theirs. As their parent or caregiver, you have made an excellent decision to look into the magic of play therapy. Using this tool, you can become a pro at understanding the big feelings in your little child and help them become a more independent person confident in themselves. You'll learn how to be your child's rock so you can guide them on their journey to adulthood with love.

This book was specifically written for parents worried about their child's development. It's for caregivers who want to help the tots in their care to get better at self-expression. It's also been written for therapists and teachers who want to know how best to work with toddlers to give them the hang of their emotions and understand the world around them. It contains therapeutic activities to help toddlers become the best version of themselves as they grow and develop.

To make this book easy to use, all the processes described here are written in a simple and easy-to-understand way. You will see the importance of play in helping your toddler naturally express themselves clearly and confidently. Discover a treasure trove of creative ideas for your toddler to play their way to a full and rich life. Everything in the following chapters will facilitate your toddler's physical, mental, social, and emotional development.

Chapter 1: The Magic of Play

If you could peek into your little one's mind, you'd be amazed at what goes on in there. It's sad that many people don't pay as much attention to their children's minds as they do everything else. You must consider your child's mental health as seriously as you do their body, and there's no better way to help them process their emotions than through play therapy. So, what does this mean? Do you just let your child go out to play? Is that it? Then, after that, do you send your children to therapy to lie down on a couch? What exactly is play therapy, and how do you use it to help children?

What Is Play Therapy?

Your toddler's mind is full of creativity, imagination, and wonder. The best way to interact with it is through the language of play. When you do that, you get to understand what your child thinks, how they feel, and what their experience in life is like. Play therapy is the gateway that allows you to enter into this world of imagination and creativity. It allows your child to express what goes in their head in a way you can understand and appreciate.

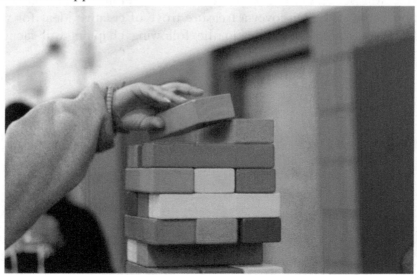

Play therapy allows your toddlers to express themselves.

Play therapy is all about letting your child fully express themselves. They deserve to explore how they feel in order to be able to understand their experiences. If you attempt to ask a child things an adult would be better at answering, you cannot expect them to respond clearly. Your child may also feel uncomfortable as they struggle with the complex concepts you present and ask them to unravel. Play therapy is a better alternative as this is a non-intrusive way to gently coax them into revealing their inner thoughts and workings. Play is the language of children. Children live in a make-believe world where imagination is not contained or constrained.

The Purpose and Benefits of Play Therapy

Your child stands to benefit a lot from play therapy. It places them in a world carefully created to allow them to play without any constraints. In this sort of environment, your child feels safe. They can wildly and freely release their innate creativity and dive deeper into their inner world. To understand play therapy's benefits, you must take a holistic look at your child's life. Think about your child as a four-part being: physical, emotional, cognitive, and social.

Play therapy allows your toddler to express themselves physically in a way that contributes to developing their gross and fine motor skills. Gross motor skills are necessary for the proper functioning of the entire body. They are responsible for standing, running, walking, sitting, jumping, kicking, lifting, etc. Fine motor skills like writing, threading a needle, and tying shoelaces require precision and control. With play therapy, your toddler will learn how to coordinate their hand movements with the visual information their eyes and brain offer them. They'll become aware of their body, the space around it, and how to move confidently through it. They'll also learn how to use their hands to write, draw, hold things, etc. They must partake in play because this is how they encourage the connections in their brain. This way, they can also develop confidence when it comes to interacting with the environment around them.

Now, onto their emotional health. Play therapy lets your toddler express all feelings and emotions, whether negative or positive, in a safe space. It allows them to externalize all their emotions so they can effectively process them. When working with play therapy to encourage emotional expression, it could involve creating a story, setting up a challenging event for your toddler to figure out, or using role play where they can feel like they are in charge. They get to feel like they have the power to explore their emotions and process them effectively. When they have the chance to express their feelings using the language of play, they become emotionally resilient and better able to handle the ups and downs that inevitably come with life.

Next, consider your toddler's cognitive health. Play therapy is an excellent tool to encourage them to develop their intellect. Engaging with their imagination and setting up scenarios where they have to solve problems or make decisions allows them to cognitively thrive. This indirectly encourages them to have flexible thinking, to come up with their own unique ideas, and to reason their way through any situation or scenario in which they might find themselves.

With play therapy, you'll also be improving your child's memory and language skills. You encourage them to tell stories as they chat freely with the therapist while getting them to think about the possible meanings of the stories they create. By working with these cognitive processes, you'll find your toddler increases their mental capacity. This makes it so they have an excellent starting point for all intellectual and academic goals they have in the future.

Finally, consider your toddler's social ability. If you want them to learn how to interact with others, they've got to develop interpersonal skills. Play is the perfect tool to help them learn the social norms and rules of etiquette that guide interactions in society. As they play, they grow confident in their ability to connect with others and maintain the relationships they find. Face it: Relationships are complicated and require more flexibility in thinking and emotional intelligence than a child may have. Therefore, engaging your child in play therapy makes it easier for them to understand what relationships are all about. They'll figure out when to negotiate, when to cooperate, and when to recognize that they're dealing with a difficult individual. You can have your child participate in group therapy or cooperative play with other children to learn the importance of sharing, waiting their turn, and respecting other people's boundaries. In this situation, you create a microcosm of society for your child to explore and understand. By doing this, you help them realize who they are, how to regulate their emotions, and how to connect with others healthily while respecting their personal boundaries and those of others as well. For these reasons and many more, play therapy is absolutely essential for your child. It is essentially a form of therapy that uses play to help your child discover and deal with psychological, emotional, and social challenges.

Real-Life Applications of Play Therapy

Play therapy can help your child deal with difficult emotions. For instance, imagine that your 5-year-old has lost their pet. It's tough for them to understand that they will never see it again. Death, as a concept, doesn't make much sense to your child, and loss is a heavy burden to bear. Engaging your child in play therapy makes it easier for them to learn the skills necessary to calm and ground themselves to heal. You can give your child a small toy representing the pet to make things easier. You can even recreate situations that remind them of the fun that they had with their pet. This might seem like a way to conjure up bad emotions, but it will offer your child a form of catharsis and teach them how to honor those they lose. They can learn to safely express grief and allow themselves to process the trauma of loss, all while holding on to the memories of their pet.

Next, imagine that your daughter has trouble integrating with others in kindergarten because she feels deep anxiety that holds her back from connecting. With play therapy, you can set up a situation for her to learn what it means to safely interact with others. Scenarios meant to explore the ideas of conflict, conflict resolution, friendship, and so on can be set up to teach her the intricacies of interacting with others from a place of kindness and empathy. These skills are necessary for her to learn so she can manage her social life and become confident enough to interact with anyone. She'll learn that the rejection of others is not a reflection of who she is.

Imagine another situation where you have a child dealing with trauma, perhaps one resulting from abuse by previous caregivers. With play therapy, you encourage these children to come out of their shells and to get in touch with what they need. The therapist guides the child to tell their story in a comfortable way while giving voice to all the ugliness within. For instance, the therapist may offer the child colors, paint brushes, and a blank canvas, encouraging them to use the art supplies and express what they feel inside. Usually, the work created by the child is an accurate reflection of their feelings, and not only that, but it also serves as an outlet for the traumatic pain that they deal with on the inside. The more your child is encouraged to express themselves in this way, the better they will deal with the trauma and pain. After this, they can move on to healing and becoming whole, healthy beings.

Building Empathy and the Parent/Caregiver-Child Bond

Using play therapy, it is possible to encourage a stronger, better connection between a child and their parent or caregiver. First, play therapy allows your child to exist in an environment that is safe and supportive of who they are. It's a pity that most children cannot simply be themselves. Sometimes, parents have the wrong idea of good parenting; other times, these children live in abusive, unsafe environments. With play therapy, the therapist works to keep your child in a playroom filled with all sorts of art supplies, toys, and anything else that makes it fun and safe for your child to fully and freely express themselves. This will offer your child a much-needed sense of security, which is essential for successfully navigating life as an adult. Also, having them feel safe and secure will make them feel much better about opening up to you because they now understand that they can create this feeling within themselves and not have anyone else take it from them. As your child plays in this environment, you are welcome to observe and even participate when you feel it's right. That will give you a unique perspective on your child's world and how you can better interact with them.

Secondly, play therapy is also essential for building trust between you and your child. Mentally healthy people can empathize with others. It's the ability to understand what someone else is going through that makes it possible to cultivate trust in all relationships. Trust and empathy are irrevocably linked. Trust lets you connect with your tots and understand them better. So, during play therapy, the therapist acts as a trusted figure and uses active listening empathy to get through to your child.

It's easy for your child to trust the therapist because the environment in which they will be playing is deliberately crafted to elicit a sense of safety. Also, play therapy involves being well attuned to everything about the child, from the words they say to the actions they take, as well as the things that remain unspoken. In this environment, your child understands that it is fine to express everything they feel because they know they will not be judged. They learn to let go of the self-consciousness that keeps them trapped in their own heads. By mirroring what the play therapist does with your child, you can also create this bond with them. You can teach your child that you are to be trusted, and they will eventually open up to you. This will further enhance the connection you will share.

By allowing children to express how they feel using play, you teach them that it is safe to be their emotional selves. Unfortunately, in certain families, children are not allowed to fully express their emotions because often, the adults in their lives are not comfortable with the truth. However, by using play therapy, you teach your child that their emotions are valid and should be expressed fully and freely.

The final point to consider when working to enhance the bond between your child and yourself is that the language of symbolism is a major tool in play therapy. It is an excellent way to uncover the truths that your little one carries within, which would unlock their personality and give you a clear understanding of who you're dealing with. Your therapist has been trained to deduce your child's various experiences, how they feel, and how they perceive the world. The more your child works with these symbols, usually dolls and toys, the more you will find yourself understanding how they process things.

Symbolic play involves the representation of actual situations in life that your child may have experienced or will experience. It gives them the chance to handle that situation in a safe space. Using this, you can show them that there's always a way to face those situations, no matter how impossible it may seem. You can use a doll to represent someone they care about, like a parent, a friend, or even themselves. Doing this gives them the emotional distance required to process what they're feeling and express it freely. You can observe their choices, the stories they lean towards, and how they react emotionally as they engage in this symbolic play to get to know them better.

Play therapy is an excellent way to discover your child. The more you learn about them, the more empathy you have for them. Also, children are incredibly perceptive. The fact that you're taking the time to understand how their mind works tells them that you care. This encourages them to lean into the empathy that you're demonstrating. Your child will get the sense that, finally, someone understands them. Someone sees them for who they are and actually hears them. This feeling is vital to developing a healthy psyche, which will help them thrive as adults.

So, now that you understand what play therapy is all about and how beneficial it can be to you and your child, the next chapter will show how art and nature can help your child unleash the creativity that lies within.

Chapter 2: Art and Nature: Unleashing Creativity

This chapter will explore how you can work with nature and art to help your toddler be creative and expressive. Understanding nature and art is essential before diving into various activities meant to help your toddler flourish. You'll also understand why these activities have been chosen, and you'll be able to adapt them as needed to make them more effective for your child. Keep in mind that every child is different. Your child will have certain likes and dislikes that you must consider and adapt to as needed.

Why Art and Nature Matter

When it comes to play therapy, art and nature are necessary. First of all, art allows your child to express themselves fully. Children do not fully grasp verbal language and may, therefore, be limited in how they express themselves. So, using art, you can skip the difficulty of asking your child to express how they feel and instead let them express themselves using sculpting, painting, and other art forms. Art allows them to visually express their internal experiences, thoughts, and emotions. It's a great way for them to navigate the more complicated feelings that even adults still struggle to process. It's also a gateway to the unconscious aspects of their psyche and will allow you to understand what goes on in their head and what they need at any given time.

Art also matters because children get to work with metaphors and symbols to show you what they're going through. By looking closely at the meanings of these symbols, you, the therapist, and your child can all work together to figure out their emotional and psychological state of being.

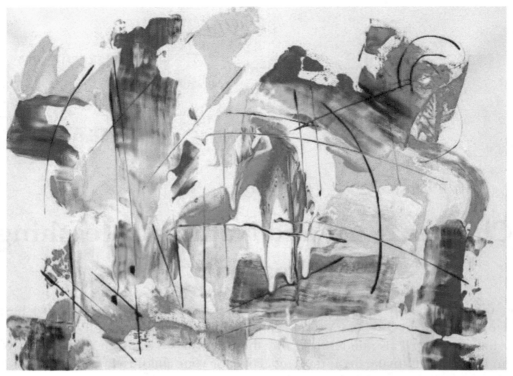

Art can allow you to figure out your toddler's emotional state.
https://unsplash.com/photos/5MTl9XyVVgM?utm_source=unsplash&utm_medium=referral&utm_content=creditShareLink

Nature is as essential as art because of the many sensory experiences that your child can enjoy. Your child will naturally feel calm and relaxed by interacting with flowers, trees, water, and other natural elements. This state of being is essential for them to express their feelings or get in touch with them. The beautiful thing about nature is its rich and multi-layered environment with all sorts of smells, sounds, colors, and textures that will engage your child's senses on every level. By getting your toddler outdoors, you allow them to connect with the world around them and feel a sense of being part of something bigger than they are.

Nature can also provide metaphorical language that you can use to understand where your child currently is on their emotional journey. For instance, the changing of the seasons could serve as a mirror for how your child feels. Winter may be an excellent way to express the concepts of loss or sadness, while spring can represent hope or feeling energized. By speaking with your child about nature and how it presents itself, your child may use what they learn about nature to express their feelings and better understand their emotional challenges. The next section of this chapter will discuss various activities you and your toddler can engage in. Some of these will be art-based, while others will be nature-based.

Art Activities

Finger Painting: Finger painting is a lovely art activity for your toddlers because they get to enjoy expressing themselves creatively as much as they want. On top of that, they'll enjoy various sensory experiences by working with the paint. Here are some of the materials you'll need for a fun finger painting session:

- Non-toxic paint of different colors

- Large, thick sheets of paper

- A disposable table cover. Alternatively, you can use newspapers to keep your work surface clean.

- Old clothes or a smock for your child to wear

- A damp towel or wet wipes to clean up after

Steps

1. Pick a good location for this activity. You can either set up an area of your living room for art or use a dedicated playroom. Your toddler should be able to move freely with no limitations.

2. You have to take care of the work surface. The last thing you want is paint stains. So, set down your disposable table cover or newspapers to keep the work surface clean.

3. Set up your work materials. The finger paint should be in containers that your toddler can reach easily. You can also use squeeze bottles instead. Set up the large sheets of paper on your work surface. You must ensure your toddler has all the room needed to make hand prints or whatever else they want to make.

4. Now, it's time to introduce your toddler to the activity. Sit them down and explain that you're both going to finger paint. Engage them by showing how stoked you are about the activity you're about to do together. You should also speak to them about it in a way they can understand. The goal is to show them you're excited so they can mirror your excitement and get into the activity with gusto.

5. Begin by demonstrating what your child should do. Place a finger into one of the colors and then stain the paper with it. If you prefer, you could plunge your whole hand into the paint because that would look more exciting to your child and encourage them to try it.

6. Now, let your toddler begin painting. Let them dip their fingers freely into the various colors to make swirls, prints, and any other shape they like. Resist the urge to give specific instructions or to demand that they do things a certain way.

7. As you paint with your toddler, get them to explore what it's like to touch the paint. Get them to notice how it feels on their hands, its texture, and its temperature. By doing this, you contribute directly to their sensory development.

8. As you work with your child, you should positively reinforce their efforts by praising them. Praise them for the colors they pick, the unique shapes they make, and how enthusiastic they are about the whole process. The more you encourage them, the more confident and expressive they will be.

9. Be open to allowing them to experiment. Suppose your toddler decides to dip a foot in the paint and use that instead of their hands. Don't stop them. Allow them to explore their imagination freely.

10. Remain in an open-ended conversation with your toddler as they paint. You should ask them open-ended questions. For instance, you can ask them what the paint feels like, what they like about their art, how they feel about what they're creating, and so on. The point here is to have a

conversation encouraging them to express themselves and reflect on their actions and feelings.

11. When the fun and games are over, it's time for you and your toddler to clean yourselves up and put things away. Help your toddler clean their hands with a damp towel or wet wipes. It's also a good idea to display their art in the end. Don't forget to tell them how proud you are of their work.

Playdough Sculpting: This is an excellent activity for your toddler because not only will they get to explore their creativity, but they will also enjoy various sensations as they work with their hands. Here's what you need:

- Non-toxic playdough in different colors. You can use a homemade version or buy some from the store.
- A work surface like a tray or a table
- Child-safe sculpting tools like rolling pins, cookie cutters, and so on

Steps:

1. Pick a good location that has adequate lighting and is comfortable.
2. Make sure the workspace is clean and safe. You may want to use a plastic tablecloth for easy clean-up.
3. Set up the various colors of playdough for your toddler. If you don't want to buy some from the store, you can create your own using flour, salt, water, and food coloring. Ensure you've got enough so your toddler can feel free to sculpt whatever they please.
4. Explain the activity to them using language they understand to get them pumped about the activity and sustain their interest and attention.
5. Begin by showing your toddler a few basic techniques for working with the playdough. For instance, you may roll it into a ball or create simple objects like snakes or triangles. Make sure that these demonstrations are simple enough for them to replicate.
6. As you work with your toddler, get them to talk about how they feel about the process. Get them immersed in the sensory experiences they have working with the playdough. Also, continue to encourage them for everything they create. Asking open-ended questions about what they're making or how they feel about what they're making is a good idea.
7. Playdough sculpting is an excellent way to boost your toddler's fine motor skills. So, show them how they can use their fingers to poke and pinch the dough. Show them how to shape things using rolling pins, cookie cutters, and other plastic utensils to give their sculpture more detail.
8. When you're done, congratulate them on doing a good job, and help them clean up with a damp towel or wet wipes. Remember to store your playdough in airtight containers or Ziploc bags for next time.

Collage Making:

These are the materials you need:

- Tissue paper, yarn, fabric scraps, feathers, magazines, colored paper, glitter, and other collage-friendly materials
- Child-safe scissors (these should only be used if your toddler is ready for them)

- Child-friendly glue or a glue stick
- A large cardboard or a large piece of paper

Steps

1. Once your space is all set up, explain to your toddler what you'll be doing together. Show them all the materials and explain all the different textures and colors. Get them to talk about how they feel about the textures they'll be working with to engage them. Remember to use child-friendly language and hype them up about what you're going to do.

2. Let them know that they have different options and don't have to stick to any one thing. Let them choose the materials they want.

3. Now, it's time to show them how to work with the child-friendly glue by demonstrating it. Make sure that you explain this process as you do it and that your language is clear and easy to understand.

4. Allow your toddler to enjoy exploring all of the materials. Let them touch and experiment with them however they want. They could tear them, cut them into different shapes, or work with them as they are.

5. As they work, encourage them to explore the sensations, congratulate them on what they're doing, and help them reflect and express themselves using open-ended conversations. When they're done, you should ask them why they chose certain things, what they love about their work, and so on.

6. When it's clean-up time, help your toddler tidy up themselves and put up their collage somewhere prominent to remind them of their accomplishment and to demonstrate to them that you are proud of them.

Sensory Bin Exploration: Sensory bin exploration is a great way to engage your child's senses. It's also good for emotional regulation. Here's how to go about it:

1. Prepare a sensory bin. In this bin, place all the things you know will give your toddler a sensory treat, like dry beans or water beads. Whatever material you choose to put in the bin must be safe for your toddler.

2. You can add other things to your sensory bin, such as little toys or objects from nature, like unique stones. Add objects that your child would be interested in.

3. Introduce your child to the activity, and explain to them that they will use their hands to feel everything in the bin. Tell them they should keep everything in the bin and be gentle as they play with the objects.

4. As your toddler feels around the bin, encourage them to notice the differences in textures, pour things through their hands and fingers, scoop things, and dig to discover the hidden items. Let them talk about what they feel and see, and teach them how to use words to express their different emotions and sensations. This is how you help them with language development. You should also be engaged in the play and show them you're enthusiastic and curious about the materials in the bin, too. You can do this by asking open-ended questions as you interact with them, making them feel supported and eager to play with the materials.

5. Encourage them to use their imagination as they play by creating various stories about the objects they find in the bin.

6. When you're done, encourage them to reflect by asking them questions – and pay attention to how they react. Take notice of what words they use as they speak with you, and pay attention to whatever else they're communicating with their body language and facial expressions while exploring the bin.

7. Now it's time for you to clean up the materials and put them back in the bin if they spilled out.

Scribble Drawing: Scribble drawing can help your toddler refine their fine motor skills while encouraging them to express themselves. Here's how it works.

1. Get all the materials required, such as crayons, markers, and paper. Make sure you have a variety of colors for your toddler to choose from and that the materials are safe for their age.

2. Choose a good spot that has adequate lighting.

3. Explain to your toddler what you're going to do, and do your best to use language that they find exciting.

4. Start off by showing them what to do. Just scribble something on the paper with markers or crayons, demonstrating how they can create various shapes just by moving their hands and wrists.

5. Hand your toddler the marker and let them do things on their own. Let them understand what autonomy feels like by encouraging them to choose the colors they want to use and applauding their choices. Resist the urge to control them or give your input.

6. While your toddler scribbles, observe them and ask open-ended questions so they can express their feelings.

7. Ensure you continue praising your tot for their efforts and creativity. When you're done, take time to appreciate what they've done. You can even go a step further and ask them to tell you more about what they created.

8. When you're sure your toddler is done doodling or it's time for a different activity, put away the materials.

Nature Activities

I-Spy

1. You and your toddler need to be out in nature for this activity.

2. Begin by explaining how the game works. You need to describe the things that you see and have your toddler spot them.

3. You start by saying, "I spy something red," or "I spy a tall blade of grass." When you say this, your toddler should look for whatever it is you "spy" and point it out.

4. Now, it's your toddler's turn to spy something.

The benefit of this is that it sharpens their observational skills, improves their language skills, and gets them to connect with nature.

Nature Scavenger Hunt

1. For this, create a list of things you can find in nature. For instance, you could add a pine cone, a soft leaf, or a rough rock to your list.

2. Show this list to your child, and head out together to look for the items and collect them.

This activity encourages your child to explore more and sharpens their senses.

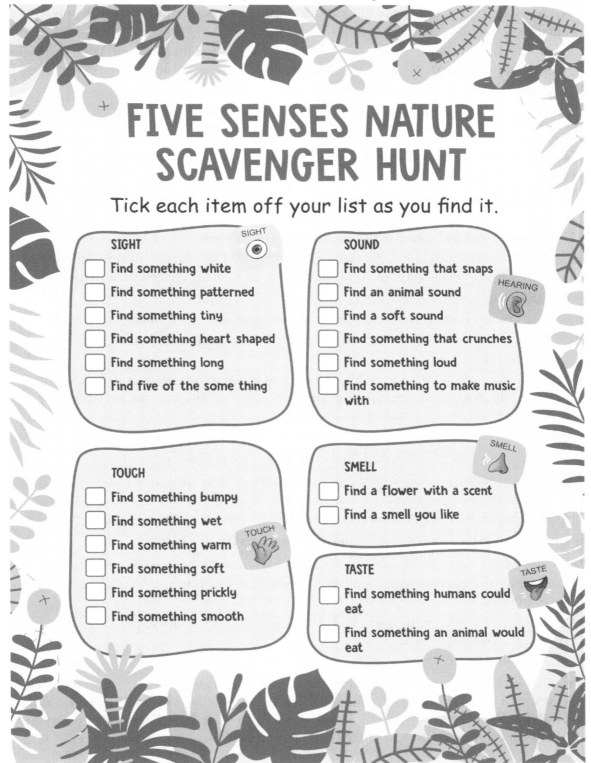

FIVE SENSES NATURE SCAVENGER HUNT

Tick each item off your list as you find it.

SIGHT
- [ ] Find something white
- [ ] Find something patterned
- [ ] Find something tiny
- [ ] Find something heart shaped
- [ ] Find something long
- [ ] Find five of the some thing

SOUND
- [ ] Find something that snaps
- [ ] Find an animal sound
- [ ] Find a soft sound
- [ ] Find something that crunches
- [ ] Find something loud
- [ ] Find something to make music with

TOUCH
- [ ] Find something bumpy
- [ ] Find something wet
- [ ] Find something warm
- [ ] Find something soft
- [ ] Find something prickly
- [ ] Find something smooth

SMELL
- [ ] Find a flower with a scent
- [ ] Find a smell you like

TASTE
- [ ] Find something humans could eat
- [ ] Find something an animal would eat

Playing with Mud

1. To avoid making a mess, do this outside the house. Set up an area with mud, some safe containers, and other utensils.
2. Your job here is to encourage your child to play with their imagination. You could encourage them by showing them how to make mud pies or an imaginary meal.
3. Make sure they don't get carried away and actually eat them.

Doing this will improve your child's creativity, imagination, and fine motor skills.

Collages

1. Gather natural materials such as twigs, flowers, leaves, branches, stones, etc.
2. Get some paper and glue for you and your toddler to use to create the collage.
3. Model the behavior you want them to copy by showing them how to tick the materials on the paper.
4. Let them arrange and stick the materials however they want.

Making collages with your child is an excellent way to boost their creativity and get them to explore their senses. They'll also feel a sense of accomplishment after having created their masterpiece.

Playing with Petals

1. For this, you need to get different colored flowers and bowls or containers.
2. Next, you and your toddler must sort the petals into different colors, placing them into different containers or bowls.

By doing this, you will help your child get better at recognizing colors and improve their sorting skills. You'll contribute to the development of their fine motor skills, and not only that, but you'll also encourage them to engage more with nature.

Playing with Sensory Bottles

1. Get some clear plastic bottles and fill them with leaves, pebbles, or sand.
2. When the bottles are filled, seal them as tightly as you can. You don't want your toddler opening them up.
3. Hand them the bottles and allow them to roll, shake, and have fun with them.

This will let them explore the various sounds and textures of each bottle.

Nature Painting

1. Use natural materials like twigs, pine cones, and leaves as brushes. You'll also need paper or a canvas to paint on.
2. Dip them yourself in some paint and hand them to your toddler. Let them dip their natural brush in the paint like you did.
3. Paint something on the paper, and encourage them to copy you or paint whatever they want.

This is different from regular painting in the sense that your toddler will be inspired by nature itself. As a direct result of engaging in nature painting, you'll notice your little one will get better at using their fine motor skills. You'll also fan the flames of curiosity in their little heart as they become a little researcher and experimenter who loves to tell you about what they've learned or noticed.

Rock Painting

1. Head out into nature with your toddler. Make it somewhere with loads of interesting rocks.
2. You can either collect as many smooth rocks as possible or have them do it.
3. Gather them all up in a pile.
4. Get some paint and markers, and let them go wild coloring the rocks.

Nature Storytelling

1. You and your toddler need to find a nice, comfortable position outside.
2. If other people are involved, get everyone to sit on the floor in a circle.
3. Next, encourage your toddler to pay attention to their environment while you tell them a story using the various objects around you in nature.

As you do this, you encourage your child to use their imagination. You also show them how to observe and improve their language skills.

Taking a Texture Walk:

1. For this, you and your toddler must take a walk in nature.
2. As you walk, encourage them to touch various natural surfaces like rocks, flowers, grass, tree trunks, etc.
3. As your toddler touches these surfaces, encourage them to share how they feel about them.
4. Let them talk about the ways the textures vary from one another.

The activity is great for improving a toddler's tactile awareness and helping them develop the necessary language to explain textures. In turn, this will get them to express difficult feelings and emotions.

Remember that for all these exercises to work, you need to always encourage your toddler to open up by asking them open-ended questions about how they feel. You can always relate different aspects of your chosen activity to their emotions. For instance, you could have your toddler hold on to a relatively rough rock and ask them what they think it would feel like to be a rough rock.

Chapter 3: Recognizing Toddler Behaviors

This chapter will explore the various factors responsible for why your toddler acts the way they do. To do this, you must first understand various theories of child development. There are a number of them, including attachment, cognitive, behavioral, and stage theories. However, some are more popular and better studied than others. As a parent, you need to have a rich understanding of these developmental theories so you're never at a loss for what's going on with your child. Everyone evolves with time, and they are no exception to the rule. These theories highlight what to expect from your child regarding how they feel and think and how they interact with the world.

Studying the way humans develop is a deep and layered topic. Everyone develops, but it's not easy to discover *what drives that development.* What makes your child act the way they do, and might that have something to do with how old they are? Does it involve the early relationships to which they have been exposed? Some psychologists say that children are born with unique temperaments, so you may wonder, could your child have a predisposition to behave in specific ways regardless of their social and environmental contexts? Developmental psychologists work hard to determine the answers to these perplexing questions to better understand a child's mind and explain or even possibly predict how your little one will likely act in their entire lifetime. This is the main focus of child development theories.

Freud's Psychosexual Developmental Theory

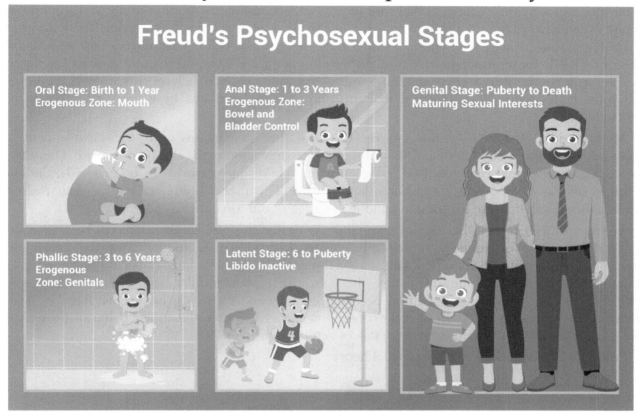

Freud had a rather interesting take on the development of a child. He did a lot of work with patients who were struggling with mental health, and in the process, he realized that how people act depends on the unconscious desires they carry and the experiences they had as a child. Freud believed that all sorts of conflicts happen in the various stages of life, which will inevitably affect your behavior and how you express yourself.

The psychosexual theory emphasizes that a toddler's development is expected to play out in stages. The developmental stages are rooted in whatever part of the body brings them the most pleasure and are expected to come with challenges that help children develop fully. Freud believed that the libido or sexual drive moves through various erogenous zones as the child moves from one stage of development to the next. If they do not successfully pass through a stage, this could result in them becoming fixated on the particular stalled point of their development. He believed that this is the reason adults act the way they do. In a situation where your child completes every stage of the developmental process successfully, odds are they will grow up to be a well-rounded individual.

Freud believed that when these conflicts aren't properly handled at each stage, the odds of the child successfully navigating what it means to be a grown-up would be slim to none. Fortunately, other development theories indicate that your child is not doomed and can actually change. As far as Sigmund Freud was concerned, there's no chance your child will be the same at age 50 as they would be at age 5, as there's no way they could continue to evolve.

Behavioral Child Development Theories

Behaviorism is a school of thought that rose to prominence in the first portion of the 20th century and would eventually become a prominent force in the field of psychology. According to behaviorists, psychologists must only pay attention to what they can observe before claiming to be true scientists. Regarding the behavioral perspective of child development, it is believed that all humans are the way they are as a result of their environment. Some of the more popular behaviorists were B. F. Skinner and John B. Watson. They believed that the only way to learn was by using reinforcement and association.

All behavioral theories operate on the premise that interactions with the environment are responsible for how a child acts, and these theories are only about what can be observed. There is no postulating or guessing what could be going on in the child's inner world. In other words, the child develops only as a response to punishment and reward. This theory holds that a child is shaped only through the stimuli they are exposed to and the language of reinforcement.

As you go through the other theories, you'll discover that this one is quite different because it does not hold any regard for emotions, thoughts, or feelings. Instead, it's just about the way the environment affects your child and vice versa. Looking at development through this lens, classical conditioning, and operant conditioning are the only ways through which your toddler can learn. With classical conditioning, they discover how natural occurrences are connected to prior events that they would otherwise consider neutral. With operant conditioning, they learn to adjust their behavior through the tools of reinforcement, repetition, and the risk of getting punished.

Erikson's Psychosocial Developmental Theory

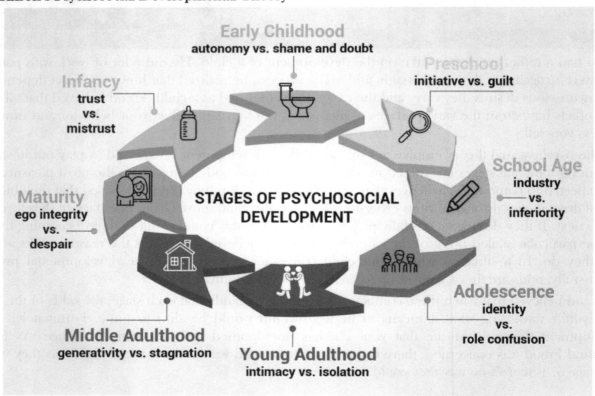

Not every psychologist necessarily agreed with Freud's take on development. Some would go on to develop their own ideas, and among them was Erik Erikson. In his theory of psychosocial development, there are eight distinct stages that properly encapsulate how people grow and change throughout their lives. These stages focus on social interaction and the various conflicts that come up at all these stages of development.

As far as Erikson was concerned, the only thing that matters is how your toddler views life and their various meaningful interactions as they go about meeting people and connecting with them. He didn't just assume the only years that matter are from ages 0 to 5, choosing instead to track toddler development from the womb to the tomb, so to speak. He also acknowledges that the unique conflicts attendant with each stage of development are crucial, as they'll affect your toddler's disposition later in life.

Bowlby's Attachment Theory

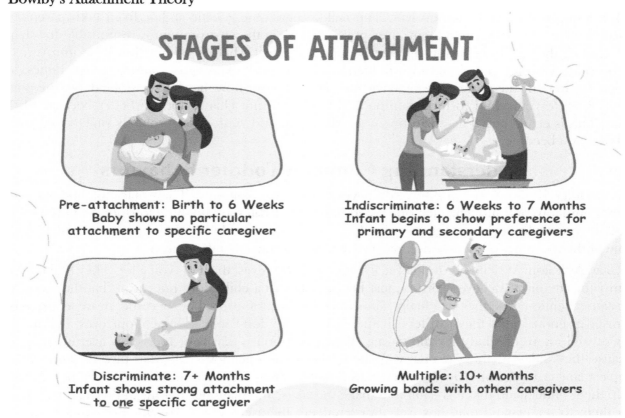

John Bowlby was more concerned with the social development of the child. He had one of the earliest theories on how this works, and he believed that the early relationships a child experiences are critical in the way that they develop throughout their life. His attachment theory indicated that children have a deep desire to be attached to others. These bonds are deep and powerful.

Think of them as invisible strings connecting you to your child, assuring them they're protected, loved, and always safe with you. You're both engaged in a dance orchestrated by nature itself, where you ensure you're always within arm's reach. Your child wants nothing more than to stick to you like glue, seeing you as their champion and hero who keeps them safe and lets them explore life around them.

Bowlby could tell that when this connection is honored by both the child and the caregiver, the little one enjoys a secure attachment style that does wonders for them in later years. However, with children who haven't been fortunate enough to have caregivers who are always present and ready to support them, their attachment style is anxious, avoidant, or ambivalent. These things will go on to affect the toddler's life as an adult profoundly, *and not in good ways.*

These are just a few of the numerous theories of child development available. As a parent or caregiver, it would be useful to learn more about these theories so you can begin to understand where your child is developmentally and what you need to do to help them make progress.

The Role of Genetics in Child Development

Child development is a dance between the environment and the child's genes. Some suggest that it is only the genes that affect the way a child develops. However, it is obvious that nature and nurture are both relevant to how the child evolves. The child inherits the genetic coding from both parents with instructions on how to express themselves physically, while the environment is responsible for shaping and crafting the child's behavior. The genes can also affect whether or not they'll be introverted or extroverted. Despite genes' obvious influence on physical expression, among other things, it is impossible to deny the power that the environment holds over how the child is molded. So, the point is to not relegate your child to the assumption that they cannot change for the better because of their genes. This is erroneous. The environment in which you find yourself is absolutely vital to who you are and who you become.

Understanding Common Toddler Behaviors

Your toddler is slowly growing towards having their own opinions. They may not understand the various emotions and thoughts that one could have, but if you took the time to study and observe your toddler, you would begin to decipher why they act the way they do. With that said, it's time to look at some of the meanings of their body language and the tantrums that they throw.

Gaze Aversion: When your toddler actively avoids your eyes, that tells you a lot. They'd like a break from your attention. Believe it or not, just because they're a child does not mean that they want your constant attention. As they gradually approach the age of two, they become more conscious of themselves enough that they can feel shame. When they don't want to meet your eyes, that tells you they're well aware of what they did wrong. When you notice that your toddler is averting their gaze because they did something wrong, you should help them acknowledge what they've done with the simplest language possible. Do so as gently as possible. Help them see how they can fix their mistakes. Help them understand that it is natural to make mistakes, and that does not mean they're a bad person. Get them to understand that they can always redeem themselves by correcting the damage they may have caused or expressing remorse for their actions.

Needing to Sleep with Stuffed Animals: When it's nighttime, your toddler wants to feel as safe and secure as possible. So, you may notice that they have a whole bunch of stuffed animals around them to feel protected. You see, your child has an active imagination that is great at envisioning monsters beneath the bed or in the dark corners of their room. This active imagination can also fuel their nightmares. Therefore, to feel at ease enough to fall asleep, your toddler will surround themselves with familiar and comforting objects, believing that they will be a form of protection against the monsters they perceive in the dark.

So, the proper thing to do is validate your toddler's need for safety and comfort and remind yourself that just because the monsters are imaginary, it does not mean they are any less real or scary to your toddler. Allow them to choose the comforting things they'd like to take to bed. Toddlers enjoy the process of making decisions, so you can ask them which books, toys, and animals they'd like to take with them. If you're concerned that they're taking too much with them, you can put a cap on how many they can take.

Hiding Their Face in Their Shirt Around Unfamiliar People: Believe it or not, just like adults, toddlers can struggle with social anxiety. You'll notice this by the various hiding behaviors that they demonstrate. This is because they don't understand how to navigate the process of socializing and dialogue just yet. They would rather console themselves using various physical and sensory expressions. You'll notice they keep tugging at their clothes to distract themselves and will even chew on them. Sometimes, they'll grasp you tightly with that infamous grip strength that toddlers inexplicably possess – likely because you represent their anchor when they are floundering in the deep blue sea of socialization. To soothe their nervous little heart, they may suck on their thumb like it's the most delicious candy they've ever had. When they're feeling really shy and nervous, they'll cover their faces using their shirts because the way they see it, if they can't see you, you can't see them, and that thought brings them immense comfort.

The way to handle social anxiety is to be gentle about it. Encourage your little one to break out of their fortress. Usually, they always look to you to figure out how they should react when they find themselves in an unfamiliar situation. So, think about what your body is telling them. If you're a bit tense, consider taking a deep breath and then exhaling to relax your shoulders, putting a smile on your face, and actively engaging with new people. Your child will model this behavior. It also helps if you use nonverbal language, such as giving your child a nice reassuring rub on their back or a squeeze on their shoulders to ensure they understand they're safe. Do not expect your child to immediately warm up to anyone they meet. Your part in all this is just to be patient with them and wait for them to warm up.

Hiding When They Poop: This tells you that your toddler would like some space and time for themselves to do their business. They do this because they have observed the adults around them doing the same thing. This is good because it tells you they're ready to be potty trained. You'll also realize that, at this point, they are very vocal about having their diaper changed. Usually, toddlers become ready to use the bathroom when they hit ages two and three. Respect their desire for privacy, but don't attempt to force them to use the bathroom just yet. All you have to do when you start to notice this behavior is guide them to the bathroom.

They Throw a Tantrum: When your toddler is acting out and throwing tantrums, they're trying to tell you they don't feel like themselves. Usually, this is not easy to deal with because it's often a shock to see your baby acting like something out of a horror movie. However, you don't have to be afraid. Just because your 2-year-old throws a tantrum does not mean this is who they are. It's simply their way of communicating with you to let you know that they need attention, are tired, or are simply bored. You have to attune yourself to what your toddler feels.

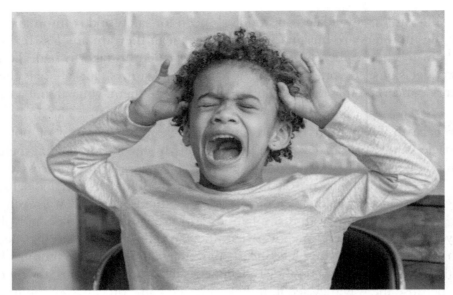
Toddlers usually throw tantrums because they don't feel like themselves.
https://www.pexels.com/photo/desperate-screaming-young-boy-6624327/

When dealing with tantrums, most parents attempt to reason with their toddlers, but this is not the time for that. Often, attempting to be rational with your toddler is useless. Instead, you must figure out what is the actual cause of their tantrum and let them know that you are aware of how they're feeling, even if you don't fully understand. You must do all you can to validate their emotions because this is what will lead them to calm down gradually.

The Tantrum Continues Even After They Get What They Want: If you're dealing with a situation where they continue to act out even after they have got what they wanted, you must remember that you're dealing with someone who's naturally impatient. They're still a baby. They don't quite understand what it means to delay gratification just yet. At this age, your toddler wants instant fulfillment. You need to be firm and not immediately give in to their needs. Instead, let them know that you have heard them out and will give them what they want in due time. This is an excellent opportunity to teach them to be patient, and with time, you can increase how long it takes between them expressing their desires and you fulfilling said desires. That is how you teach them to be patient.

Being Possessive When Other Children Are Around: Sometimes, your toddler exhibits clingy, possessive behavior, and it's difficult to understand why. This tells you that they think they don't have your attention or not enough of it. You can bank on this being the case if you've been a little too busy recently or if there's a new baby in your home. When there haven't been any changes in how you've been spending time with them, or there's no new baby, odds are that this possessiveness simply indicates that they are becoming increasingly aware of themselves. It's a phase where children become obsessively possessive of their parents, but you must understand that's not bad. It tells you that they are starting to become aware of their personhood. At this point, they identify themselves as being connected to the things that have the most value to them, and as their caregiver, you are at the top of that list.

So, how do you handle a possessive child? You should give them a hug. Let them know that, yes, you definitely are their parent or caregiver. Express to them in no uncertain terms how much you love them. You can also take advantage of this by teaching them about the importance of sharing. You can tell them that you are their parent, true, but it is okay to be kind to other people.

Activities to Understand Your Little One Better

Shower your toddler with affection and encouragement. When you show your child affection, you demonstrate tenderness and love to them. You show them warmth in your interactions with them. How do you do this? First, you begin with physical touch. Touch is the primary language children use to begin understanding the world around them. So, little things like kisses, hugs, holding hands, cuddling, or rubbing their backs could comfort them. When you do these things, they feel like you love them, and they feel safe and secure.

Eye contact is another excellent way to demonstrate affection to your toddler. As you speak or play with them, always look in their eyes warmly. Eye contact is a nonverbal way to let them know that you have your full attention, whatever they're talking to you about matters.

Affection also implies quality time every day. You could read a book with them, talk about their day, or play with toys. The important thing is to be present. Some parents assume that spending time with their children means being in the same room while doing their thing, but that's not right. Turn off the television and put your phone down. Your child should have your full attention as you actively engage them.

Also, listen attentively and actively to your toddler. Do what you can to understand them, respond to them, and remember what they tell you. It doesn't matter how trivial what they're saying appears to be. Remember that it means the world to them in their little heart.

As for encouragement, don't just praise your toddler when they get something right. Praise them for also putting in the work. Praise them for their effort. If they tried to draw a chair, and it didn't turn out like a chair, you can commend them for trying and being creative rather than reprimand them for making mistakes.

Encouragement means celebrating the small wins, like when they finally learn how to tie their shoelaces or decide to share with a playmate. As you encourage your child, you create an environment where they can safely express themselves. You allow them to do things for themselves instead of taking away a learning moment by doing it for them. You act as a support and assist as a guide to them while you allow them to take charge. By offering support, you encourage them to feel confident and independent. Also, never compare your child to another because that would damage their self-worth and inhibit their abilities and personal growth.

Make a habit of reading to your child every day. Reading with your child is more than a bedtime routine. It's an opportunity for them to learn, develop emotionally, and connect with you on a deeper level. Consistency matters, so set aside a specific time for your child to read with you daily. Having a specific part of the house dedicated to reading is helpful. Make it nice and comfortable so you're child always wants to be there when it's time.

Don't keep reading the same book to them. Instead, have a diverse selection. The books should vary in topics and styles and suit your child's age. You can make reading fun by taking your child to the library and letting them pick the books that they're most interested in. As you encourage them to read, you help them develop cognitively, and their language skills improve. Since most stories have moral lessons, your child can learn about ethics and values, which will help build their character. You also foster a spirit of curiosity within your child.

Show your little ones how to express themselves in healthy ways when they're upset. Emotions are unavoidable. They're part of being human. Your child will begin demonstrating emotions at a young age. So, giving them the tools they need to manage and express how they feel healthily is a great idea. This skill isn't something people are born with. It's an ability that is learned.

So, how do you teach your child how to express themselves? First, you must model healthy expression. Your child watches you keenly and will act the way you do. When you're upset, speak clearly about your feelings calmly, breathe deeply, and resist the urge to be hostile.

Encourage your child to talk about their feelings by talking about yours. You can tell them, "I felt upset that time..." or, "I felt relieved when..." It's great when children see that everyone has different emotions and that it's okay to feel how they do. Validate your toddler's feelings by listening to them actively and not dismissing them. To comfort their children, some parents say things like, "It's not a big deal" or "Don't cry." Never discourage your child from crying if that's how they feel. Instead, you could say, "I can tell you're not feeling so great right now. How about we talk about it when you feel like you can?"

Another way to teach your child to handle their emotions healthily is to show them different coping mechanisms, such as breathing exercises. Show them how to count to 10 when everything feels too much. Teach them to use art to express themselves. Have them go outside and get active to release their emotions through running, jumping, shaking, or anything else. Role-play situations where you and your child act out different emotions and how to respond to them in various contexts. Rather than only comfort your child, teach them how to make empowering decisions to feel better at the moment.

Set boundaries that are appropriate for their age. Boundaries are essential because they help your child feel safe and secure and give them structure. They understand why certain behaviors are necessary and know what is expected of them and what to expect from them. Your child may not be able to carry a glass of water at their age safely. So, a reasonable boundary would be using a safe sippy cup until they accomplish the physical milestone where they can safely carry a glass of water.

If your child is younger, they may be unable to express their more complex emotions. So be patient with them and give them the tools that they can use to tell you how they feel. Those tools include the necessary vocabulary or charts displaying emotions in a fun way. Remember what your toddler is capable of in terms of cognition. You can't expect a 3-year-old to be okay with waiting for something for a long time. So, rather than criticize them for impatience, you can find ways to distract them.

Whenever you set a boundary with your child, give them choices. It doesn't help just to tell them no. If they would like to have some candy before dinner, you could give them the option of a healthy snack or choosing what they'll have for breakfast the next day.

Whenever your child respects and follows boundaries, positively reinforce compliance by appreciating them and offering them a reward. Also, explain the rationale behind the boundaries you set. Your child may not understand why it's not okay to hit or bite. By letting them know it's not okay because it hurts other people, they're more likely to respect those boundaries in the future.

As your child grows, you can allow the boundaries to morph with them so that you account for their increasing capabilities and offer them more freedom and responsibilities. You can let them decide when to go to bed or what to wear out. You can also work together when creating rules so they don't feel you're just giving them orders.

Model the social skills and emotional skills you'd like your toddler to have. Children copy the older ones in their lives who have more experience of being on earth than they do. Give them the correct blueprint to follow. Show them what it's like to be calm in the face of stress or intense feelings. Demonstrate how to actively listen, share and take turns, and behave politely. Show them the importance of owning up to mistakes and apologizing when it comes to conflict. Teach them how two people can devise a satisfying solution when faced with a disagreement.

Teach them empathy by acknowledging how they feel when distressed or pleased about something. Show them what it means to be kind. As you demonstrate these behaviors, narrate them to your child. Let them know why you do what you do, and they'll model that. Whenever you slip up (and you will, because you're human), show them what it's like to self-reflect. If you raise your voice at someone, you can say, "I was upset, but I shouldn't have raised my voice. That was wrong of me. Next time, I'll handle my emotions better and be kinder."

Chapter 4: Role-Playing — Perception and Empathy

This chapter will show various engaging role-playing activities to help your toddler understand and express their emotions.

The Importance of Role-Playing Games

Role-playing games are vital when it comes to developing empathy and being able to take on other perspectives. As you role-play, your child has a challenge set before them. They need to take on a different persona, which makes it possible for them to develop empathy as they understand other people's feelings and thoughts and can appreciate someone else's perspective.

With role-playing, you can teach your child to put themselves in someone else's shoes so they can see how the world works through new eyes. This is essential for developing empathy. Empathy is vital for socialization, and it's a skill that your child needs to learn if they're going to stand a chance of developing successful social connections and handling conflict effectively and productively.

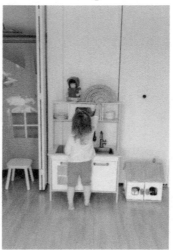

Having your child role-play will encourage socialization.
https://www.pexels.com/photo/cute-toddler-girl-playing-with-toy-kitchen-at-home-3933230/

You can use certain games to help your child get in touch with their emotions, practice socializing, and learn how to effectively pass across their point of view to other people while being respectful. So, when you encourage your child to take on a different persona or perspective, you offer them the opportunity to understand themselves even more and understand others.

Understanding Empathy

Empathy has two aspects to it: the emotional aspect and the cognitive aspect. Emotional empathy is being able to experience what someone else feels emotionally, while cognitive is being able to imagine what someone else is dealing with emotionally. For instance, if your child sees that their friend is in tears, emotional empathy will move your child to want to help this person out. However, suppose your child is only working with cognitive empathy. In that case, they only understand that the other child is dealing with sadness and needs to be comforted somehow. Cognitive empathy is something your child will get used to much later in life, as your child understands they have a much different perspective and experience than others.

Empathy matters because your child needs to learn why rules matter and what makes something right or wrong. Not only that, but they will also discover behaviors that are beneficial to socializing, such as assisting others. Empathy will help your child successfully navigate their social life, an intricate part of being human. On top of that, your child will enjoy quality relationships that last long as they master empathy.

Teaching Your Child Empathy

When you want to teach your child how to be empathetic, you must serve as a role model by being warm and caring. Odds are they will act the same way with other people. Also, you should teach them to understand their emotions better and label them appropriately. Remember, being empathetic relies heavily on the ability to experience someone else's feelings or imagine what they may be going through. Therefore, you cannot escape teaching your little one about emotions; this is how you can get them to become empathetic. Labeling emotions and explaining what emotions feel like will make it easier for them to understand how others feel and be concerned about those who aren't having a good time.

You must validate every emotion your child feels, even when it is uncomfortable. Unfortunately, certain parents would rather minimize their children's feelings. They never allow them to express themselves and choose to shut them down before they can even get a word in edgewise. Don't be this kind of parent. You must explain that how they feel always matters. Help them understand that just because someone else feels differently does not automatically mean their own feelings are invalid. Show them that you care about their feelings, and you're essentially modeling excellent, empathetic behavior for your child to copy.

You also have to be okay with letting your child know how you feel at any point in time and why you feel that way. Emotions can be tricky and complicated things for a child to understand. That is mainly why toddlers choose to throw a tantrum instead of communicating what's bothering them. When you take the time to express how and why you feel a certain way, you're modeling behavior that encourages your little one to turn within and do some introspection. You also make it easier for them to rely on their intuition because they understand that their feelings are not to be dismissed. They will learn that they must recognize the causes of their feelings. This will do wonders for your child later on when they're an adult interacting with others who may be manipulative or have ill intentions.

Role Playing Games

1. **Emotions Charade:** With this game, your child can play with you or with a group of other children. One person acts out emotions while the others are left to understand or try to guess what that person is portraying and feeling. This is an excellent way to engage your child and have them understand how emotions work. Here are some emotions to consider: happiness, sadness, boredom, anger, and excitement.

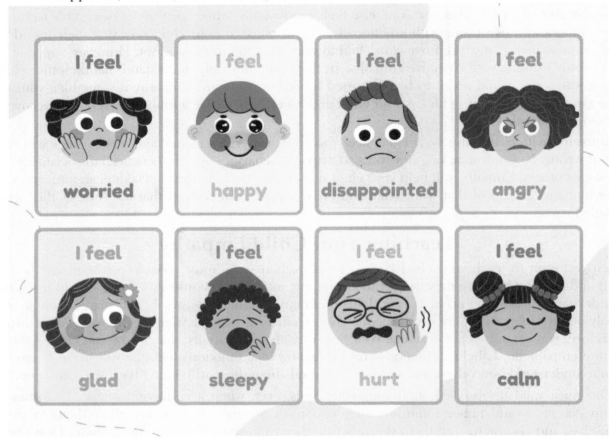

2. **Family Role Reversal:** With this exercise, your child can pretend to be other family members, such as a sibling or a parent. The idea is to work with their imagination. Your child is meant to take on the various responsibilities and tasks connected to the people they're portraying. By taking on different family roles, your child is better able to understand the responsibilities on everyone's shoulders and be empathetic towards them.

3. **Puppet Show:** In this game, you and your children should use puppets to try to express different real-life situations and the emotions attached to these situations. This will help your child learn how to communicate clearly and creatively. Real-life scenarios could include being in a position to help someone else, comforting someone who has lost a pet, dealing with a sore loser, and so on.

4. **Story Role Swap:** This game involves seeing the world through someone else's eyes. You and your child should take turns telling a story from various characters' perspectives. You

could work with any story you want and get creative with it. You can use real-life stories or work with fairy tales.

5. **Animal Adventures:** You and your child will take turns acting like different animals, thinking about how the animal might feel in various scenarios. This is great for helping your child learn empathy, even towards animals. It's also a good way to help your child learn respect for wildlife. They can learn what it means to feel as powerful and dangerous as a lion or as fragile as a bird.

6. **Helping Hands:** In this game, there are two roles: the helper and the one being helped. You and your child need to take turns acting in these roles. As you do this, your child will begin to understand the importance of reaching out to others to help, as well as asking for help when something gets to be a bit too much.

7. **What Am I Doing and Feeling?:** This game involves copying each other. Start off by performing facial expressions or movements and then letting your child copy you. Then, you can let your child take the lead. This activity results in your child becoming more attentive to people around them, and they learn how to deduce the implications of other people's actions and choices.

8. **Mirroring Emotions:** By playing this game, your child has to figure out what the faces you make mean emotionally. So, this implies that your child must understand the various emotions one could experience before they can successfully play. When your child gets it wrong, you can just help them understand by explaining.

9. **Drawing Faces:** With this exercise, your child should draw various faces that demonstrate different emotions. They don't even have to be good at drawing. They simply need to get the basic attributes of a face. As your child draws, you can engage them in conversation about what it is that could make someone feel whatever emotion they're depicting.

10. **Empathy Drama:** In this game, you and your child will take on different personas and even dress the part to reenact scenarios. As for characters that you may want to play, consider the various people who don't have an easy time of it at school or at work. So, think about the new child in school, the painfully shy one, the one who gets picked on, the one who is always alone, and so on. You can have your child play each of these roles and then have them play themselves while you take on the roles. As you play, you should ask them how they feel when they portray any of these characters, what they'd like to do to help them, or what they'd prefer others to do in that situation.

Tips for Supporting Your Child During Role Play

- Do your best to remain present and engaged as you carry out these activities.
- During each of the previous activities, don't forget to model empathy.
- Encourage your child to think about the things they learned from each activity.
- Always offer your child positive feedback for trying, and encourage them whenever they feel challenged.
- Make sure that the environment in which you role-play is safe so that your child feels comfortable expressing or trying things they've never done before.

Chapter 5: Applying Attachment Theory

People have always sought to understand the causes of development in terms of emotions. As a result, a certain theory that closely examines childhood's early days has been developed. This theory is known as the attachment theory. In the early days of childhood, the child's heart is fragile, and their soul is only just budding, becoming a fully-fledged human being. The attachment theory seeks to explain the process of the child's development emotionally.

Attachment theory sheds light on the emotional bond between the child and their caregiver. With this theory, you have a vivid picture of how human relationships work, as it captures emotions such as love, the idea of trust, and the importance of security, which all come together to form the child's sense of self. These elements will act as the blueprint for how your child will interact with everyone else as they mature.

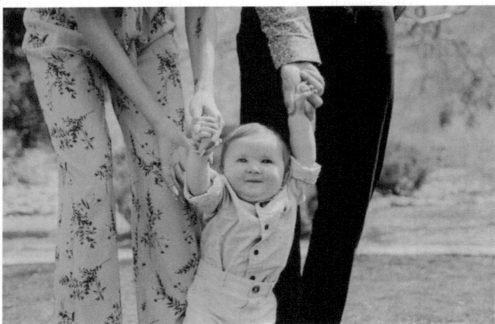

Children tend to be attached to their caregivers.

When it comes to play therapy, the attachment theory shows how to help your child develop healthily regarding their emotions. When your child has the space to play, it opens up their heart so they can show you what they truly are afraid of, what they're curious about, and what it is they desire from life. By working with play, your child can set off on a journey of discovering who they really are, and attachment theory acts as their North Star, showing them the way to their authentic self.

The Basics of Attachment Theory

This theory, developed by John Bowlby, posits that all the relationships and interactions you and your little one share will profoundly impact how the child develops emotionally, socially, and cognitively all through their life. According to this theory, your child desires to be as close and connected to you, the primary caregiver, as much as possible. You act as a base of security from which your child can head out to explore the world and return to you when they need to be comforted or reassured that everything is fine.

Another aspect of attachment theory is attachment behaviors. Your child will show specific behaviors meant to help them remain as close to you as possible so they can continue to enjoy your care and love. Among these behaviors are smiling, reaching out for you, cooing adorably, or crying. These behaviors are essential because they help the toddler survive. Not only that, but when they are responded to appropriately, they help your toddler develop a secure attachment to you.

There are also attachment styles to consider. According to this theory, your toddler will develop an attachment style that depends on their experiences with you. There are three main attachment styles to consider. The first one is the secure attachment, where your toddler feels securely attached to you in the sense that they are confident you will always be there for them. They know that if they reach out to you, you will respond. Because they know this, they feel safe heading out into the world, knowing that they can always come back to you if anything goes wrong.

The next style of attachment is known as the insecure avoidance attachment. When a toddler has this attachment style, they don't really care whether or not they are separated from the person who's supposed to care for them. They don't demonstrate much in the way of distress and will usually either avoid the caregiver or ignore them completely.

The final attachment style is the insecure, resistant, or anxious attachment style. Here, the toddler demonstrates very clingy behavior. If your child is this way, you'll notice that they're very anxious. Whenever they're not with you, they become very distressed. However, when you return, they're lukewarm to you at best as they both want to be comforted by you all while resisting it.

The Importance of a Secure Attachment Style

A secure attachment is essential because it will allow your toddler to become emotionally secure. This attachment style contributes to the development of your toddler's brain. Those who are securely attached tend to be more curious about life, more creative when it comes to solving problems, and generally perform better when it comes to cognitive functions.

Another thing to note about the security attachment style is that it is excellent for reducing the risk of various mental conditions like depression, anxiety, and other disorders in later life. When a child has an insecure attachment, it makes it difficult for them to navigate their emotions, and of course, interpersonal relationships become a source of pain. By choosing to understand the attachment theory, you can do all you can in your power to promote secure attachments between you and your child to give them the best shot at life, and there's no better way to accomplish this than through play therapy.

How to Foster Secure Attachment

Play therapy is necessary for creating a secure attachment between you and your toddler. For one, it creates an environment where your toddler can feel safe and trust you fully. In this situation, working with a therapist, you and your toddler can enjoy a space that is welcoming to each other and has clear boundaries so your child can feel safe and secure.

The excellent thing about play therapy and developing a secure attachment style is that it is a non-directive approach. Your child does not need to take orders, making it easy for them to take the lead. They get to be the ones to set the tone for every activity, while your therapist is only a facilitator, and you only serve as an observer. This way, you allow them to express themselves as fully and freely as they want without interrupting or judging them. There's much to learn from simply watching the way your child plays.

To foster secure attachments, you're working with play as a language. Your child may not be able to understand much else, depending on their age, but they do understand what it means to play. Thanks to play, they can express their emotions and thoughts, and they can share their inner experiences with you in ways that are easy for them. Children do not yet have the language necessary to paint their inner landscape in terms of emotions and thoughts. Play is a great way to encourage them to do this, which will, in turn, ensure a secure attachment between you and your toddler.

Part of fostering a secure attachment is allowing your child access to various therapeutic tools and materials that excite them. Among these are puppets and dolls, and there are art supplies and other objects that could be of symbolic importance to them. The idea is to offer as many things as possible that allow the child's imagination to feel free and roam wild. By doing this, you encourage your children to be themselves and feel that you are their safe space.

During play therapy activities, you and your therapist should actively listen to your child, paying attention to the various ways in which the child expresses themselves through play and the words they choose to share their thoughts. The therapist is engaged in reflective listening in the sense that they will reflect everything your child is sharing back to them to validate their emotions. This will lead to the development of empathy. You can mirror this behavior at home to encourage your child to feel securely attached to you.

Using play therapy, you can encourage secure attachment by teaching your child emotional coping skills as well as regulation skills. Using play, your child can learn how to figure out what they're feeling and then healthily express those feelings. They can learn how to identify when they're out of sorts and use various techniques to help them control themselves.

Play Therapy Activities to Foster Secure Attachment

1. **Puppet Time:** This activity involves you and your child playing with dolls or puppets. You should take turns playing different roles, such as the child or caregiver. This way, your child will understand empathy and communication, and you both understand each other, which is conducive to developing a secure attachment.

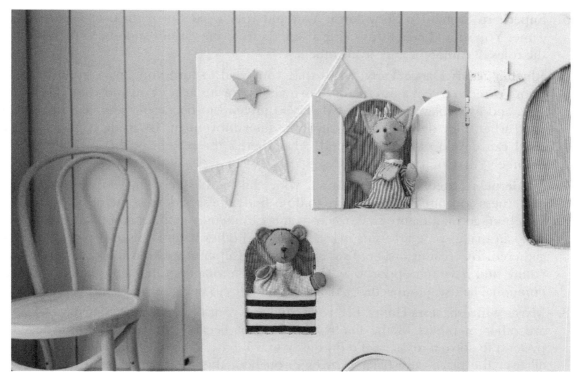
Playing with puppets can help your child form a secure attachment.
https://www.pexels.com/photo/close-up-shot-of-a-puppet-show-7356596/

2. **Team Adventure Quest:** This activity is – essentially – anything you and your child can do together to develop your bond. This could include anything from physical activities to board games or puzzles. The idea is you want to be able to solve problems, make decisions, and collaborate with each other. Some examples of these games may include trying to solve a puzzle together, building an obstacle course or a fort and completing it together, and so on. Whatever you choose, ensure your child can handle it by considering their age and that you're both having a good time while you connect and cooperate with each other.

3. **Imagination Station:** For this game, you and your toddler pretend that you're on a train that needs to get somewhere and is powered by stories. You're going to start a story, and then you'll have your toddler continue, and then you pick it up from wherever they leave off. As you do this, you will be allowing them and yourself the opportunity to explore emotions, solve problems, and discuss the subject of relationships. All of these things will serve to increase the bond between you. When the story ends, you and your toddler can make-believe arriving at your final destination and getting off the train.

4. **Colorful Fun:** This activity is a simple one. You and your child get to pick whatever medium of art you want to use to express yourselves, as long as it involves loads of colors, and then get into it. You can discuss how you feel and express yourself as you work on your art. You can talk about various things that your child is experiencing at school, allowing them to open up to you. Working with art allows your child to connect with their emotional side, which means you understand their inner world even better and create a secure attachment to your child.

5. **Superhero Switch-Up Showdown:** You and your child can participate in this role-playing game. You should take turns being a superhero, using various superhero powers, and share the roles of caring for and saving others.

6. **Rhythm Safari Dance Party:** With this, you need to turn your living room into a dance floor. You can give it a fun theme, like animals, for instance. You and your child can dance, sing, and even play instruments while you pretend to be various animals. Encourage your child when they demonstrate creativity in their movement. By using dance, you and your child can develop a stronger bond. Also, there's the benefit of the laughter that you will definitely share in the process.

7. **Wilderness Explorers Expedition:** If your child is old enough, you can take them on a wilderness adventure. All you have to do is find a local park or some nearby nature reserve. You both go on a nature walk where you get to identify animals and plants, and at the end, you can make some art using twigs, leaves, and other natural bits and pieces that you have gathered. By creating a shared experience, you will improve your toddler's appreciation for nature and have the opportunity to communicate openly with each other to discover your emotional landscapes together. All this contributes to being securely attached to each other.

8. **Mystery Investigators Unite:** Tell your child that your home is now a detective's lair. If there are other members of the family, this is great because you can all come together and pretend to solve a mystery. To do this, you will have to create various clues, hide messages all over the place, and place puzzles throughout the house. This is an excellent game to encourage your toddler to communicate with you, collaborate with others, and figure out how to solve problems. It can not only improve the bond that you and your toddler share but also the bond between them and other members of the family.

9. **Magical Time Machine Journey:** This storytelling method will improve the bond between you and your child. You both need to take turns telling stories traversing through time and space. You and your child can create amazing scenes and sensations, relax with each other, and connect. Your story can cover anything from futuristic worlds to ancient civilizations. You could even decide to delve into the realm of magic.

10. **Cosmic Sensation Adventure:** Working with bags full of glitter, some water, and various shapes in confetti colors, you can create a sensory experience that your child will love. Both of you should explore the various sensations in this bag. You might also want to use some slime to make things even more fun. Encourage your child to squish the objects, move the bags around to form various lumps, and work with their imagination.

Practical Advice for Parents and Caregivers

- Take every opportunity to cultivate empathy by trying to see the world through your child's eyes and understand how they feel and see things.

- Be responsive to your child. Whatever their needs may be and whatever cues they give you, respond right away.

- Be consistent in your responsiveness. Responding to them one minute and ignoring them the next isn't a good idea; that's how you create trust issues and a feeling of uncertainty in your child that will plague them for the rest of their life.

- You must engage your toddler in therapy play every day. These games are about communicating with each other, sharing your experiences, and exploring the emotions you both feel.

- Always be clear in your instructions. You need to be clear about the rules of each game so that your child understands what to do and you have a better time together.

- Encourage your child to be open and to communicate with you by ensuring there's no room for them to wonder if it's safe to say what's on their mind without being put down or shut up.

- Encourage the spirit of teamwork. This will go a long way in helping your child learn to collaborate with others, solve problems, and make decisions as part of a team.

- Your little one is not too young to understand the concept of appreciation. Therefore, whenever your child's making an effort, you should celebrate that. Let them know that you see what they're doing and that they are doing great.

- Active listening is an essential skill that you can teach your child by modeling it. Not only should you pay attention to what they say, but you should also tell them that you understand by reflecting all those experiences and emotions back to them. That is how you validate their feelings to help them to be a well-rounded individual.

- Nothing should be so important that you don't get to spend quality time with your little one. You should dedicate time each day to spend with your child. That is how you encourage a secure bond with them.

Chapter 6: Sensory Strategies

This chapter will introduce various activities that will stimulate and engage your child's senses.

What Is Sensory Play?

Sensory play is the sort of play that involves stimulating the senses, including sight, touch, smell, taste, and hearing. Sensory play is necessary for your little one's brain to develop as it should. It is the basis for developing other skills, including social and cognitive capabilities.

Why Sensory Play Is Vital

Sensory play is a great way to help your child develop physically, cognitively, and emotionally. It engages your toddler's senses on various levels. Sensory experiences are a great way for them to be stimulated, providing their brain with the fuel it needs to be capable of more complex cognitive skills. By allowing your toddler to work with various colors, shapes, and textures, they'll be much better at processing information from their senses, developing better spatial awareness, and solving problems.

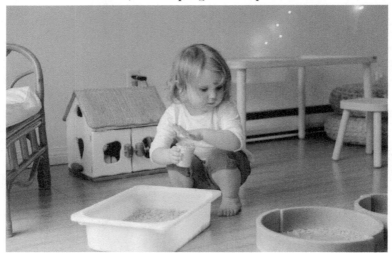

Sensory play engages your toddler's senses.

Another reason sensory play is vital for your toddler is that it helps them integrate information from their senses to understand their environment. In the future, they will be well aware of where they are, how to handle themselves, and how to stay safe. By working with various sensations, your toddler will be much better at processing sensory input and organizing that information. This will inevitably lead to a much better ability to focus for extended periods, hold their concentration on something, and regulate the way they respond to external stimuli.

Sensory play is great for your child's fine and gross motor skills and proprioceptive and vestibular systems. By engaging your toddler in sensory play, you'll notice they get better at manipulating small objects such as pens, pencils, or crayons, scooping, pouring, and squeezing materials from one container into another. All of these will inevitably do wonders for their motor coordination, and it will improve their dexterity, too. Your child's gross motor skills improve as they climb tables and trees, maintain their balance on a leg or a ledge (proprioceptive), jump from one spot to another (vestibular), etc. Not only that, your child's coordination and strength will improve.

Sensory play can also be a wonderful thing for the development of language. The more your child explores various sensory objects, the more they talk about them in conversations with you and describe their experience, then the more they'll learn how to work with words to communicate their ideas. They will understand the words related to sensations, textures, colors, and more. This is a great way to improve their lexicon and their ability to communicate.

Sensory play is great for the regulation of emotions. It offers a controlled and safe environment for your child to explore everything around them and express how they feel about it. The sensory stimuli you provide your child can stimulate their interests. It calms them down when they feel too anxious or irritable. This is a great way to teach your child how to regulate their emotions and soothe themselves when they're not feeling so great. You may offer your child a stress ball that they can squeeze whenever they're feeling tense, and you can also let them play with soft and soothing materials to allow them to feel relaxed whenever they're a little too stressed out.

Social interaction and communication are two things that are also improved by sensory play. As your child engages in these activities with other children and with you, they learn the importance of sharing and taking turns. They discover that sometimes you can cooperate with others and that when things are difficult, you can always negotiate. This will help them get better at socializing with others and being empathetic. Also, sensory play is excellent for your little one to understand other people's perspectives by choosing to collaborate with them.

Your child's imagination and creativity will soar as a result of engaging in constant sensory play. The materials you work with tend to be open-ended in nature, which means that there are so many possibilities for your child, and they can come up with so many different scenarios. They take what's just a regular pile of sand and shape it into a castle or a ball, or they could use playdough to create all kinds of things. This encourages them to think divergently and to get better at problem-solving.

Sensory play is great because every child is naturally curious about the world surrounding them. When you actively set up sensory play activities, your child gets to enjoy satisfying the desire to explore, experiment, and discover life. Through these experiences, your child will become even more wondrous about the world around them and will want to consume even more knowledge.

Different Types of Sensory Play

Various kinds of sensory play are classified according to the senses they engage. Each of them matters because they will help your child learn about the world around them and how to interact safely and enjoyably.

First, you have the sort of sensory play that requires working with the sense of touch. These activities include playing with water, sand, clay, or play dough. This will offer your child various opportunities to figure out the different textures, sensations, and temperatures.

There is also sight sensory play, which employs your child's sense of sight. This is exceptional for sharpening your child's sense of perception and cognitive skills. Among these are sorting activities, where your child arranges things according to shape or color, puzzles, or playing with shadow and light. All of these can help your child learn visual distinction and how to solve problems.

Sound sensory play will help your child's auditory perception and develop their linguistic skills. As they listen to some good music, create their own fun tunes, or play games that require listening to and making sounds, your child will become a fabulous listener, able to pick up subtle nuances that others miss in conversation. They will also develop a sense of rhythm.

Taste sensory play is a great way to help your child learn about their preferences when it comes to food, as well as all the various flavors that exist. Among these activities are baking or cooking with you to guide them, trying out foods they've never had before, or taking part in games involving taste to help your child develop a more complex palate.

Smell sensory play obviously works with your child's sense of smell. You can teach your child about the various aromas and scents that exist. You can work with herbs or spices, toddler-safe perfumes, slime, scented play dough, etc. You can also craft games based on smell where your child has to guess what it is they're smelling.

Sensory Activities

1. **Rainbow Rice Sensory Bin:** For this activity, you'll need a large container that you fill with different colors of rice. You should also provide your toddler with cups, scoops, and other small toys. The cups and scoops are meant to help your toddlers scoop up some rice and pour it. All the various toys are to be hidden within the container of rice so that your toddler can feel around for them. This will work on both your toddler's sense of touch and sight.

2. **Scented Playdough:** You can scent your playdough using food extracts or essential oils. Make sure that these materials are safe for your toddler to interact with. They can have fun shaping and squeezing the dough. This would engage their sense of smell and touch while helping them develop various skills.

Watermelon Kool Aid Play Dough Recipe

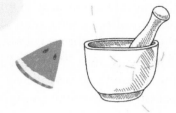

Scented watermelon playdough is easy to make and such fun watermelon activities for kids of all ages! Use in watermelon theme or summer play. (Not for Consumption)

Equipment

> 2 large bowls
> stove top to heat water

Ingredients

1 packet Watermelon Kool-aid unsweetened drink mix
1 cup flour
1/2 cup salt
1 cup water
2 Tablespoons cream of tartar
1 Tablespoons Vegetable Oil, or similar

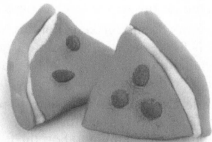

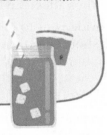

Ingredients

1. Commence by blending all the dry components (excluding the kool-aid) in a spacious bowl.
2. Proceed to bring the water to a boil on medium heat. Once it's boiling, transfer it to a bowl and introduce the oil.
3. Integrate the amalgamated dry components. Should it remain sticky after thorough blending, consider adding roughly 1/4 cup of flour incrementally. Let it cool for 5-10 minutes or until manageable.
4. Upon reaching a manageable temperature, divide the kool-aid playdough into two portions. Approximately 1/4 of the dough will represent the watermelon rind, while the remaining 3/4 will form the succulent red fruit. To avoid getting your hands messy, utilize a ziplock bag for food coloring. Apply green food dye to the smaller portion and mix.
5. Embed dry black beans into the red section to mimic seeds. Indulge in the joy of molding and playing with this entertaining watermelon-themed activity!

3. **Bubble Wrap Stomp:** With this activity, you only need a sheet or two of bubble wrap. Allow your toddler to jump and stomp on the bubbles barefoot to pop them. If they want, they can also pop the bubbles with their fingers.

4. **Sensory Nature Walks:** Take your toddler on a nature walk, but this time, the goal is to encourage them to touch everything they can as long as it's safe. Be mindful of such things as poison ivy. Have your toddler also pay attention to the various sounds of nature around them as well as different smells.

5. **Sensory Balloon Play:** This activity requires grabbing some balloons and filling them with rice, sand, or water. Allow your toddlers to enjoy squeezing and rolling the balloons, paying attention to the various weights and textures of each one.

6. **Sensory Sound Shakers:** For this, you need some small containers and fill them with such things as bells, beans, rice, and some sand. Have your toddler shake each of these containers and pay attention to the various sounds that are produced. By having your toddler do this, you teach them to discriminate between sounds, understand rhythm, and develop their fine motor skills.

7. **Taste Exploration:** This sensory play involves having your toddler taste appropriate foods for their age. You should have bitter, salty, sour, savory, and sweet things. You should have your toddler pay attention to how the food tastes and how it feels in their mouth.

8. **Sensory Painting:** Give your toddler various materials they can use to paint, such as sponges, feathers, or various objects of different textures. Encourage them to notice the differences in the textures and how the textures affect the kind of patterns that they can create with these objects.

9. **Sensory Water Play:** Provide your toddler with various containers of water with different objects of different sizes. They should also vary in terms of the shapes and textures of these objects. Have your toddler pour the water, splash around, and feel what it's like as they explore the objects within them. This way, you will improve their tactile sensation, hand-eye coordination, and much more.

10. **Ice Chipping:** For this activity, you will take some of your toddler's toys, put them in some water, and then freeze them. When they're nice and frozen, you can set your toddler up with some safe hammers so they can break the ice. Make sure that your toddler is old enough to do this safely and that you do not leave them unsupervised. It's very satisfying for them to chip away at the ice. This will offer them better hand-eye coordination, an understanding of their strength, and satisfaction when they finally get at the toy. They can also enjoy safely exploring what cold feels like.

11. **Sensory Optical Course:** You're going to create an obstacle course using all kinds of fun materials like throw pillows, textured mats, balance beams, and tunnels. Allow your toddler to climb, crawl, twist, and turn through this course. In the process, your toddler will work with their tactile sense and learn how to move their body.

12. **Sensory Sock Bin:** Grab a bin and fill it up with socks of different textures, such as silky socks, ripped ones, fuzzy ones, and so on. Get your toddler to feel around in this bin so that they can explore the various textures. Not only can they touch them, but they can also stretch the fabrics. You can also get them to sort them out based on the way they feel.

13. **Sensory Hide and Seek:** For this exercise, you're going to hide little objects or toys in a sensory bin that's filled with other stuff like shredded paper, dried beans, or rice. Your toddler needs to

dig through these materials to discover the items you've hidden.

14. **Sensory Water Beads:** Grab a container and fill it with water beads. Let your toddler have fun enjoying the squishiness of these beads and their vibrant colors. Let them pour, scoop, and transfer the beads however they want to, using their hands, cups, spoons, and other tools.

15. **Sensory Sound Walk:** Take your toddler on a walk around the block or your neighborhood. As you walk, encourage them to pay attention to the various sounds around them, such as their footsteps. Let them pay attention to what it sounds like when walking on gravel versus on grass or pavement. Get them to also feel what it's like with their shoes on one surface versus another.

16. **Bubble Wrap Painting:** Set up large sheets of bubble wrap to serve as canvases for your little one to paint on. Make sure you provide them with washable, non-toxic paint. Demonstrate how interesting this can be by showing them what happens when you pop the bubbles after painting, as it creates unique textures and patterns. This lovely activity will encourage your little one to be more creative.

17. **Sensory Story Time:** Choose one of your toddler's favorite story books, which has loads of sensory elements, like pop-ups, interactive parts, textures, and so on. Read it to them and allow them to explore and interact with the various sensations of the book.

18. **Sensory Garden:** You can create a sensory garden of sorts for your little one by getting together materials like flower petals, soft grass, smooth rocks, and scented flowers. Put them in a play area. Encourage your child to go around the garden touching, smelling, and observing the different colors and textures of each item.

19. **Sensory Obstacle Course:** You can set up an obstacle course, but this time, use materials that have very different textures, colors, and so on. Whatever you choose to include as part of the obstacle course, it's got to be something that will not hurt your child or make them find it boring. You should encourage your toddler to overcome the obstacle course and take their time exploring the various sensations and sights around them. You can also use auditory cues to make the activity even more engaging for them.

20. **Musical Charades:** Play different clips of music that represent various emotions. Play a little bit and then ask them to express what they felt as they listened to the music. If you have safe musical videos for your little one to watch, you can also play those for them and have them communicate the emotions the singers appear to be feeling.

21. **Bedtime Sing-Along:** This is a great way to have a calming routine to get your toddler to wind down for the day. It's a great activity that will help them relax and feel secure. You can just sing a song or lullaby and get your toddler to sing along with you.

Tips for Safe and Engaging Sensory Play

- Always pick material that is safe and age-appropriate for your toddler. You should avoid small objects that could be choking hazards and always look for non-toxic materials.

- You must always be nearby to closely supervise your child. Pay attention to their actions; when needed, you should intervene to keep them from ingesting materials they shouldn't or to stop an accident from happening.

- You must create a designated space for sensory play. This should be an area where your child can play and explore safely and where they understand that boundaries should not be crossed.

This will help you clean up more easily when they're done.

- You must also set boundaries in the form of ground rules. Let your toddler know what's okay for them to do, and clearly express the guidelines they need to follow.

- When working with your toddler on sensory play, make sure you're using a sensory tray or a bin. This way, you contain the area in which they play, and it's easier for them to have fun exploring the various materials you've provided.

- Think about their sensory preferences. The way to do this is to pay attention to what your child prefers. You'll know this based on the toys or materials that they tend to ignore during the sessions. In their next session, provide them with the colors, textures, sounds, senses, and tastes you know they prefer.

- Consider every sense your child has and look for materials to engage and stimulate them. You can combine music with some tactile materials.

- When your child is done with sensory play, you must always follow up with something that would calm them. This is because sensory play can be very stimulating. Therefore, consider getting your child to read a book, engage in cuddle time, or play some quiet music so that they can relax once more.

Chapter 7: Play and Socialization

This chapter will show the importance of play and encouraging social skills in your toddler.

Theoretical Perspectives on Play and Socialization

The Social Learning Theory: According to this theory, when it comes to learning and socialization, what matters the most is observation and behavior modeling. In other words, children tend to look around them to observe other people's behavior and then mimic those behaviors. This is how your child learns about the various social roles and expectations that exist.

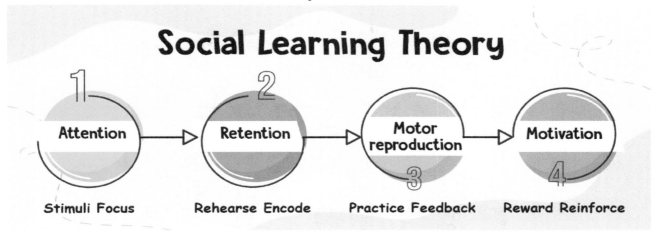

The Cognitive Developmental Theory: This theory focuses on how much play matters when it comes to a child's development and how it is connected to their ability to socialize. This theory suggests that through play, your child will be able to understand how the world functions and have the social skills necessary to connect with their peers.

COGNITIVE DEVELOPMENT

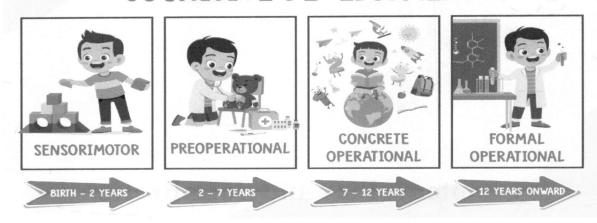

SENSORIMOTOR	PREOPERATIONAL	CONCRETE OPERATIONAL	FORMAL OPERATIONAL
BIRTH – 2 YEARS	2 – 7 YEARS	7 – 12 YEARS	12 YEARS ONWARD

The Social-Cultural Theory: This theory is about the cultural and social influences your child is exposed to and how these affect how your child plays and socializes. According to this theory, play is essential for developing cognitive and social skills.

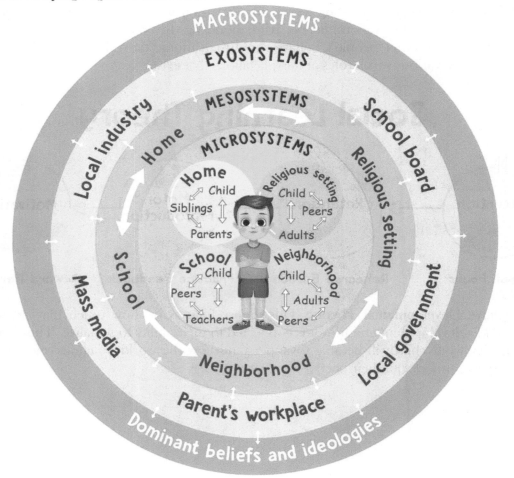

Symbolic Interactionism: This theory is also heavily centered around play in terms of symbolism. Symbolic play is all about working with various objects and specific actions to represent other things. Your child will be able to practice various social rules, roles, and languages. It's about working with their imagination so they can internalize these things and use them in their real-life experiences.

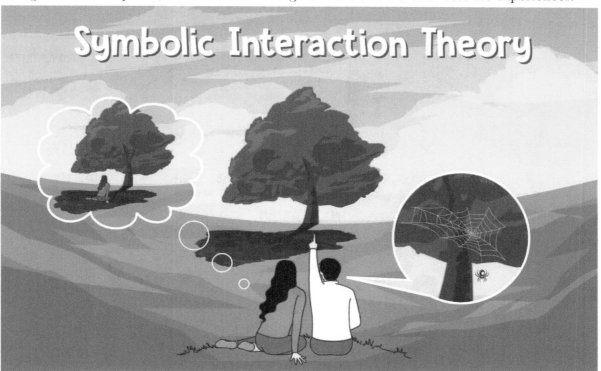

Ecological Systems Theory: This theory is about how peers, the community, and the child's immediate family can work together to influence how they play and socialize.

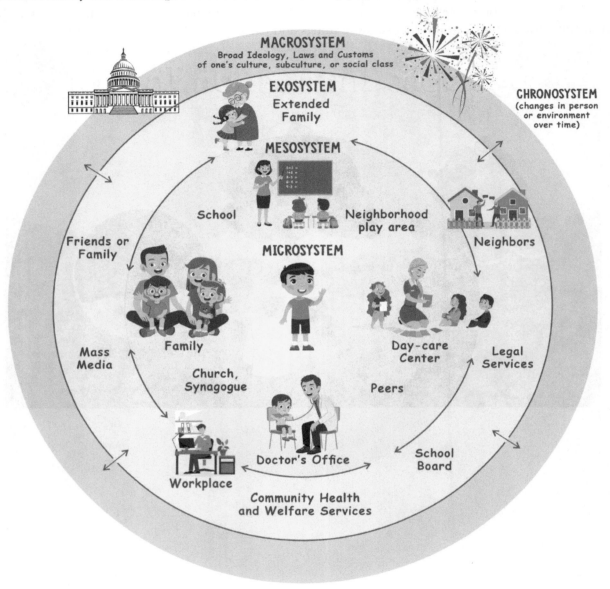

Cultural-Historical Theory: This theory is about the social-cultural influences that affect your child's ability to play and socialize and the historical influences that have led to this present point. It's about the importance of various tools of culture, such as playing materials and language, in helping your child mediate their interactions with others and how they learn about life.

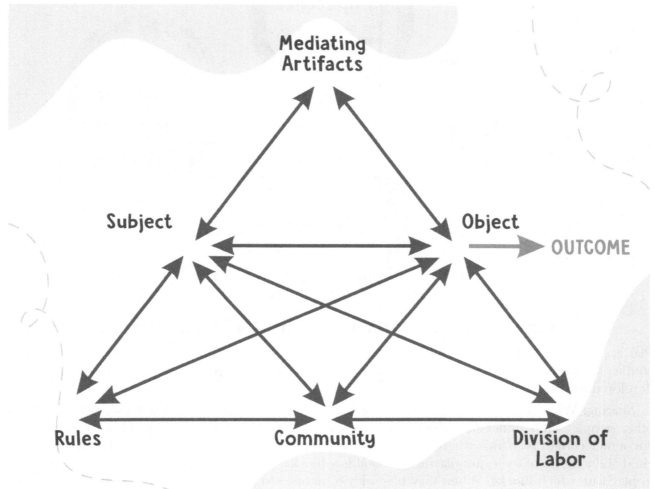

The Self-Determination Theory: This one is about the intrinsic desires and the sense of autonomy that your child has when it comes to playing and socialization. According to this theory, when your child is engaged in play activities that align with their desires and allowed to be a competent individual, your child will experience the very best situation for social development. All of these theories provide different perspectives that you could use to understand the ideas of playing and socialization and how they affect your child's life.

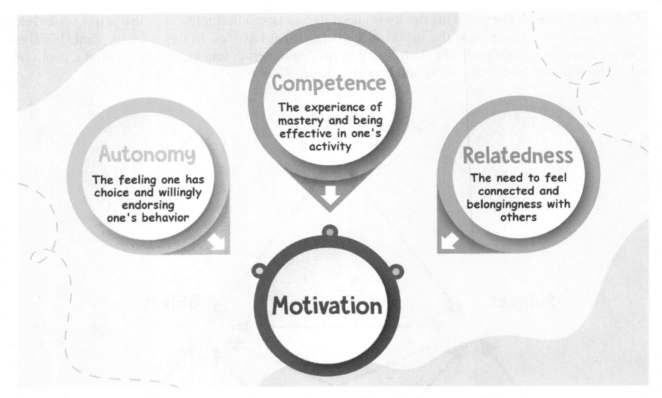

How Play Supports Your Child's Development

Play is essential to helping your child develop the skills they need to survive in life, such as cooperation, conflict resolution, and sharing. Here is a very detailed look at how you can use play to help your child develop these skills.

Sharing: When your child plays, they have the opportunity to practice what it means to share with other people. They understand the importance of having to take turns. As your child plays, they will encounter certain scenarios where they must share their toys, other materials, or roles. Imagine your child and a friend of theirs are playing with building blocks. They may need to negotiate whose turn it is to play with which blocks. When they play with someone else, your child will understand these things and learn to think about other people's perspectives and wants.

Cooperation: Play is also a great way to encourage a child to work with others to achieve a specific aim. When you and your child work together, or when your child cooperates with others in play, your child learns the importance of collaborating. They understand they cannot just take their opinions and feelings and lord them over everyone else. Your child learns to communicate effectively and to listen to what others are actually saying to them, as well as the importance of coordination.

For instance, imagine your child is part of a group of children who are working together to create a fort on the playground. Obviously, each of these children will have certain tasks they must perform, they will have to share ideas, and they must be supportive of one another if they intend to actually build that for its success. By cooperatively playing with others, your child will learn how to work as part of a team to solve problems and how to effectively communicate their wants and needs.

Conflict Resolution: The great thing about playing is that your child has a safe environment in which they can learn about conflict and how to resolve it. As children play with one another, it's natural for conflicts to come up. These are often over who gets to share what, whose ideas should be implemented, or which goal matters most. Imagine your child and another are in disagreement over which game to play next. They can both learn to negotiate and compromise and work up a mutually satisfying solution. For instance, your child may agree to take turns to play each game or come up with a different game that they both want to play right away. Through the avenue of play, your child will learn how to deal with various conflicts and come up with various strategies for resolution, such as expressing how they feel, actively listening to the other person to understand them better, making compromises, or seeking guidance from others more competent or grown-up when required.

Perspective Taking: Your child needs to learn how to take on other people's perspectives if they're going to have a chance to develop empathy and understand other people's feelings. There's no better way to accomplish this than through play. Using imaginative play, for instance, your child can take on all sorts of roles and pretend to be someone else, which would allow them to see life from other perspectives besides their limited view. Your child and others may decide to play doctor or house, and together, they can come up with different situations, allowing them to relate more easily to the feelings and perspectives of other people.

Following Rules: Play is an excellent tool to teach your younger one the importance of following rules. Society would fall apart if there were no rules. Therefore, by using play, you can teach a little one how to stick to the rules and why they should. Playing games centered around rules will teach your little one the importance of being fair to others and not breaking any rules. You can engage your little one in a board game that has various rules and involves taking turns. This has the added advantage of teaching your child the importance of patience.

Solving Problems: Playing is a great way to enhance your child's ability to solve problems as they deal with the challenges and conflicts that arise as they play with their peers. Your child will learn how to spot a problem when it crops up, brainstorm to figure out a way around it – and take stock of the results of their chosen actions. For instance, imagine your child is part of a group working on creating a bridge with building blocks, but the blocks keep collapsing. Your child and other children may then decide that it would be best to try a different approach. They know they have to devise a different strategy and work together as a team to solve the problem. As your child plays, they'll learn it is okay to try things and have them not work out how they expected. By learning they won't always get things right, they discover they can think creatively to solve problems, and they can critically analyze what they did wrong so they can get it right *the next time*. It also teaches them that there is no reason to feel bad just because they came up with a solution that hasn't worked. They just have to try something else. These are all the ways in which play can help your child in social interactions, cooperation, and negotiation with others.

Activities

1. **Pretend Play:** Engage your toddler in imaginative scenarios like playing doctor, house, running a restaurant, managing a school, and so on. By playing this way, you encourage your child to interact with others socially, learn to negotiate and communicate with others, and so on.

2. **Cooperative Board Games:** Invest in getting board games that require your toddler to work with others.

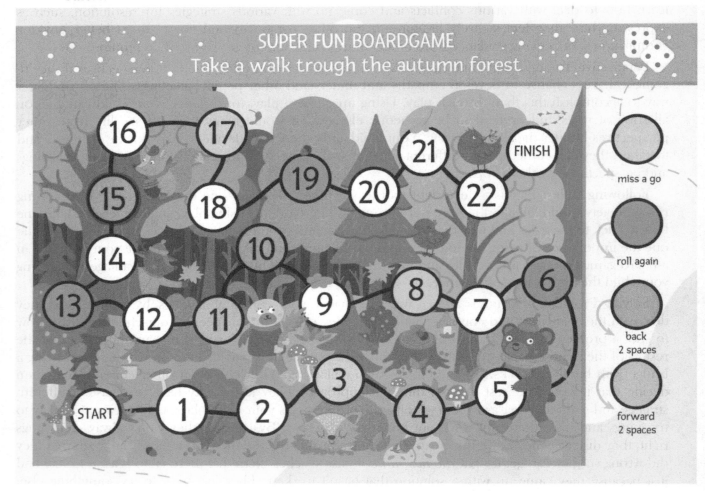

MEMORY GAME

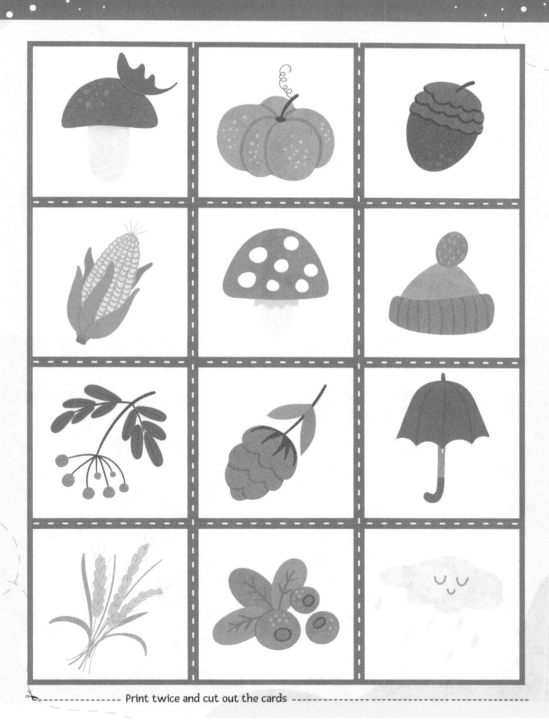

HELP THE BEAR GET TO THE BERRIES

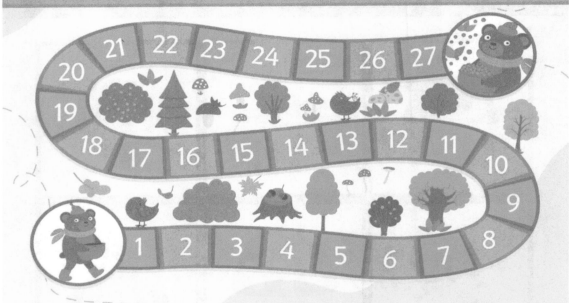

HELP THE GIRL GO THROUH THE JUNGLE

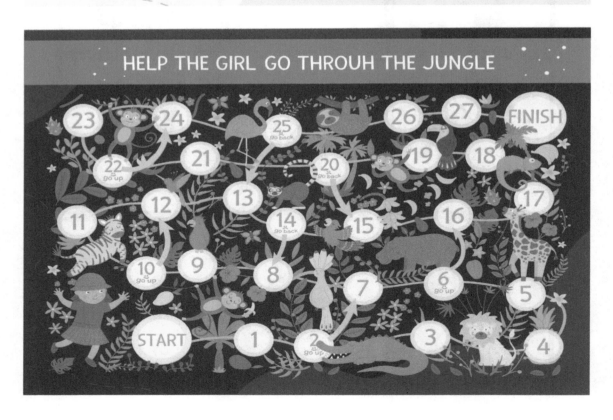

3. **Construction Challenges**: Get your toddler to work with others. You should provide them with Lego blocks, magnetic tiles, etc. You can then ask them to create something such as a car, bridge, or the tallest tower they can.

4. **Team Sports**: You can have your toddler participate in team sports, allowing them to learn the value of communicating with others and cooperating. Some of the best sports to consider would be soccer, baseball, basketball, or even relay races.

5. **Collaborative Art**: There's no reason your toddler should make art on their own. You can get other toddlers to join with them. Consider such things as collage making, mirror painting, or group sculpting.

6. **Pictionary**: Charades and Pictionary are excellent ways to allow your child to communicate with others and work to understand them. The great thing about these games is that they involve working with nonverbal cues and finding creative ways to express yourself.

7. **Puppet Shows**: You can have your child perform puppet shows with you or other children. Let them improvise. This will allow them to be creative and interact with others. You'll also teach your child inadvertently about character development, telling stories, and performing with others.

8. **Group Science Experiments**: Getting your child to cooperate with other children is a fantastic way to ensure they'll have no problems finding their feet socially the older they get. Using group science experiments is a fun, efficient way to teach your child how to get along with others, so get them involved as often as you can. Encourage your child to use their skills of observation. You can have them work with other small groups of children and carry out simple experiments such as mixing colors to see what they'll get, testing the various properties of water, and so on.

9. **Set Up Team Building Challenges**: An example would be building a bridge using limited materials. You can challenge the children to try solving a puzzle within a given time limit. This would encourage your child to work with other children to figure out the problem as quickly as possible.

10. **Circle Time**: This activity involves having children sit together in a circle to share stories, experiences they've had, or other things they enjoy with others in the group. The idea behind this is to foster listening skills, get your little one to interact with others, and actively understand what others are sharing.

Strategies to Support Social Play

Try Guided Role-Play. This is a great way for you to encourage your child to develop socially. You can offer your child various scenarios, themes, and props to play with others. You could create a pretend grocery store and have the children take on various roles so that they can communicate and negotiate with each other. One child may play the manager, another the cashier, another a shopper, and so on.

Model Appropriate Behavior. As the adult in the room, you must act in a way your little one can copy. Along with other adults, try to demonstrate to your child how to communicate effectively, share with others, take turns, and resolve any issues that may arise. You can do this by modeling how to actively listen, solve problems, and respectfully communicate disagreements with others.

Encourage Cooperative Playtime. As often as possible, always set up situations where your child can play cooperatively with others. This is essential if you want to give them a shot at being a social master.

So, sign your child up for any events or activities that will require them to collaborate with others, empathize with their peers, and work as a team to make decisions.

Chapter 8: Music and Emotional Regulation

When it comes to emotional regulation, music can have a profound effect. This chapter shows the power of music and how it can help your toddler handle their emotions.

The Connection Between Music and Emotions

Have you ever listened to a piece of music and felt like it moved your core? Good music will do that to you, as it takes you to beautiful heights and depths of emotion, helping you explore your inner landscape. It moves you. It has the power to evoke feelings you didn't even know you had. It can even impact your emotional well-being and change the way you perceive life. Music has the ability to influence your emotions because it directly influences certain parts of your brain involved in the processing of emotion, including the hippocampus, amygdala, and prefrontal cortex.

When it comes to play therapy for your toddler, music is a tool that you can use to help your child recognize their emotions and express them. For instance, when your child is encouraged to listen to all sorts of music to figure out the various feelings each piece evokes, you are essentially teaching them how to handle their emotions. You're teaching them that depending on what they're listening to, they may feel a certain way. You can even encourage your child to try to create their own music as an outlet to express the way that they feel.

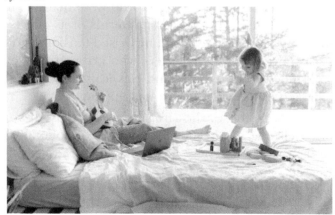

Music can help your child recognize and express emotions.
https://www.pexels.com/photo/happy-young-woman-playing-ukulele-for-daughter-at-home-3975635/

Music can help your child to develop their emotional and social skills. Engaging your child in certain musical activities involving other people, such as playing instruments as a group or singing in a choir, can help your child learn about the power of communicating with others, cooperating, and developing empathy. It is also a great way to offer your child a shared emotional experience and the feeling of being connected to other people. The human experience is one that is founded on the principle "no man is an island," implying everyone is a social creature, no matter how introverted or reclusive they are. Music, therefore, is a great unifier that can solidify the bonds your child forms with people around them.

Music is so powerful that some World War II veterans in the United States were treated using music therapy. This form of therapy had very effective results on people who struggled with traumatic brain injury, neurological conditions, and psychological issues like PTSD.

Music and Mood

The fact that music can serve as an excellent way to improve mental health is not a new thing. It's been known for several thousands of years. Think about ancient philosophers like Confucius and Plato or the kings of Israel who understood the importance of singing praises to deal with stress. Even now, military bands use music in order to boost the morale and courage of the soldiers. When you're watching any sporting event, you'll notice that there's music playing in order to make the crowds and the players more enthusiastic about what's about to happen. In schools, children work with music to help them memorize certain concepts or the alphabet. Go to a shopping mall, and you notice that the kind of music that plays is meant to lull you into a sense of comfort and make you not want to leave the store. Go to the dentist's office, and you'll notice there's some music playing to help nervous patients calm down.

Genres and Effects

There is a plethora of musical genres, and having so many options makes sense when you consider differences in personal taste, culture, the emotional tone of each genre, etc. Yet, in spite of these differences in musical genres, there are certain universal responses. Babies really enjoy the sound of a lullaby. A mother singing to her child is a very soothing thing, regardless of whether the mother has a great voice or not. There are particular genres of music that make people feel terrible even when they claim to enjoy it. In a study of 144 adults and teenagers who were made to listen to four different sorts of music, of all the genres, grunge music was the worst in terms of its effects on people. It led to a rise in hostility, made people even sadder than they were, increased tension, and caused the entire group to feel fatigued. This was the case even for the teenagers who claimed they enjoyed grunge. In another study, college students who listened to pop, rock, and classical music said that only the former made them feel optimistic about life and even made them a lot happier.

Music is also excellent for helping those who struggle with anxiety. If your toddler is anxious, you can play something relaxing. Relaxing music can regulate their emotions and improve their cognitive abilities when they're throwing a tantrum. There have been studies that suggest that music is excellent for handling depression as well. You don't have to be depressed, nor does your toddler, to enjoy music's uplifting effect. It's great for treating those with medical conditions and illnesses like burns and cancer, too; for this reason, it only makes sense that if your toddler is throwing a tantrum or struggling to grasp a concept, you can simply play some calming music for them.

Music and Memory

Another great thing about music is that it's much easier for you to remember things if you put them in a song. Music has been known to enhance your memory and recall. It is especially great for children and adolescents who struggle with attention problems. You can use it to reward them for acting in the way you'd like them to. If your toddler pays attention to something serious, like their homework, for about five to ten minutes, you may reward them with a chance to listen to some fun music for just about five minutes.

Music for Focus

You can even work with songs, interesting rhythms, and even dance to help those who struggle to focus. Working with baroque music is excellent for improving reasoning and attention. If a student is playing background music, it's not distracting for them and could help them focus as long as the music has no lyrics. You can also use musical cues to help your little one tell when it is time for one activity or another. Finally, when you play calming music, you encourage open, outgoing, and social behavior. You reduce the possibility of being impulsive.

Musical Activities

1. **Soothing Lullabies:** You don't have to be an opera singer to pull this off. If you can't sing, all you have to do is play soft lullabies to calm and soothe your toddler. There's no lovelier way to bond with your toddler than when it's time for them to hit the hay at the end of the day, and you need them to calm down because they're feeling stressed or throwing tantrums.

2. **Musical Breathing:** For this activity, you must guide your toddler to take deep breaths while playing calming instrumental music. You can model how they should breathe by showing them what to do. Factor in how deeply they're able to breathe, as they may not be able to take as deep a breath as you can. Make sure you're both breathing in sync with the music, as this is a great way for you both to relax and even increase your bond.

3. **Sensory Shakers:** Whip out the little handheld shakers and give them to your toddler. Your shaker can be full of stuff like beads, beans, rice, or dried pasta broken into pieces. Next, you're going to shake them in various rhythms. Then, get your toddler to copy. Choose rhythms that are easy to emulate. This will help them develop a sense of rhythm and calm them down.

4. **Expressive Dance:** You can show your toddler how to move, sway, or dance freely to the music they choose. This is a great way for you to work with them when they're throwing too many tantrums. They may have a lot of pent-up energy that they need to release. Moving is a great way to express those emotions and help them regulate their feelings.

5. **Exploring Instruments:** You should get a few child-friendly instruments and allow your toddler to explore them. Allow them to play however they want, no matter how bad it sounds. It doesn't matter if they're making actual music. The point here is to get them to explore the various possible sounds.

6. **Stories with Music:** Tell your toddler stories while you have some music in the backdrop. Make sure to choose music that matches the theme of the story you want to tell so you can enhance their engagement. With time, you may point out to your toddler how the music made the story more dramatic or interesting by trying to tell the story again without the music. This is a great

way to teach them that they can emotionally regulate with music.

7. **Dancing with Scarves:** Give your toddler a few colorful scarves, and play some music at different tempos. You should get them to move freely and express themselves by playing with the scarves.

8. **Musical Mirroring:** You and your toddler need to stand face-to-face. Then, while playing some music, make random dance moves and let them imitate you.

9. **Hunting for Sounds:** This exercise involves you and your toddler going around the home or outdoors to listen carefully and try to figure out the different sounds. Among the ones to look out for are the sound of the fridge humming, water running, birds chirping, trees moving, distant music or traffic, and so on. This is a great way to encourage your toddler to become more aware of their surroundings and the sounds in them.

10. **Musical Yoga:** If your toddler is old enough to control their body, you can practice some yoga with music playing in the background. The music should be soft instrumentals, and you can guide them through easy stretches. This will help them to become more aware of their body and relax even further.

11. **Writing Songs:** They don't have to be masterpieces. They just need to be written by both of you. Encourage your toddler to share their input and create melodies or lyrics based on the things that they have experienced and what they're feeling.

12. **Music and Puppet Play:** You can play some music while your toddler works with puppets to act out various stories or songs. You can switch through different songs with different moods so your toddler can change the story to match the song. By playing with puppets and using music to tell stories, you get your child to notice the structure inherent in storytelling, which means they'll get better at this skill with time.

13. **Name the Tune:** This is a lovely, fun one where you get to play snippets of songs that your toddler is familiar with and encourage them to guess the name of the song. This is a great way to get your toddler to be able to recognize sounds easily and improve their memory and knowledge of music.

14. **The Singing Ball:** In this exercise, you and your toddler can sit opposite each other or in a circle with other people. Ideally, you should have a soft ball. Pass it back and forth or around the circle as you sing a song together. This is a great way to encourage your toddler to learn the importance of waiting their turn, interacting with others, and enjoying time with others.

15. **Musical Hide and Seek:** For this game, hide a toy somewhere in the room and then play some music to help your toddler find the object. The closer they get, the louder the music should get. The further away they are from the object, the quieter it gets. This is a great way to encourage them to pay attention to what they hear, get better at spatial awareness, and solve problems.

16. **Transitional Music:** Work with music that is rhythmic and upbeat to encourage your toddler to be excited. This is the kind of music you should play to start the day. By using music to mark when it's time to switch to a different activity, you'll reduce the odds of them arguing with you or getting fussy about having to stop whatever they're doing. Music is also an excellent tool for grabbing your little one's attention, so that's a bonus you can take advantage of.

17. **Create a Mood-Based Playlist:** You should have a playlist of songs for certain moods. Take the time to curate a playlist that will have various effects on your toddler, like getting them hyped up

or calming them down.

18. **Musical Freeze Dance:** You will need to play some energetic music. The idea here is to get your toddler to dance however they want, no matter how goofy it looks. Every now and then, you're going to pause the music, and when you do, they will need to freeze in a pose. This way, you'll be teaching them how to listen, control themselves, and regulate their emotions.

19. **Singing Feelings:** When your toddler feels down or excited, you can get them to sing about their feelings. Certain songs already address these different emotions, such as "If You're Happy and You Know It" or "If You're Angry and You Know It." Alternatively, you can get your toddler to freestyle and just sing about how they feel. You don't need them to sing a particular melody, as the goal is to just let them do what they can and have fun with the game. It is a good idea for you to model this first to give them the confidence to copy you.

20. **Drum Release:** If you offer your toddler some drums or percussive instruments, you can get them to let go of whatever negative feelings they're having. Banging on drums is a great way to get rid of pent-up anger, frustration, and tension. On top of that, they'll have so much fun that they end up tiring themselves out in the end.

21. **Relaxation Time:** This activity involves playing calming, soothing music. The music should not have any lyrics that will distract your toddler and make them excited or agitated. You may want to play these when it's time to relax or calm down. Or, you can help them focus on their homework or whatever activity it is they're doing by playing this relaxing music.

22. **Emotional Humming:** This is almost like singing feelings, except that, in this case, you are going to encourage your toddler to hum to express how they're feeling at the moment. So, first, get your toddler to identify the emotion they have before humming about it. As usual, you should first model the behavior so they know what to do.

Chapter 9: Evaluating Progress and Overcoming Challenges

The Importance of Regular Progress Assessment

You should regularly assess your child's progress when it comes to play therapy. You must understand that for your child, play therapy is a great therapeutic outlet that helps your child communicate and express themselves just as they're naturally inclined to. Play therapy is a safe and supportive way for your child to explore their various emotions and take responsibility for their actions. Not only that, but play therapy will also help your child solve their problems more efficiently.

You must realize that as a parent, you have a very important part to play in supporting your child's progress. You can't just hand over your child to the therapist and expect that everything will work out. You must be actively involved, and part of that means you must regularly check in on their progress.

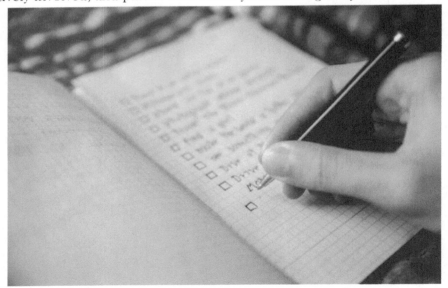

Progress assessments can help you see how your child is developing.
https://unsplash.com/photos/RLw-UC03Gwc?utm_source=unsplash&utm_medium=referral&utm_content=creditShareLink

Give yourself some homework: To learn about your child and study them as you would study a new subject you don't understand yet. The more you learn about your little bundle of joy, the more you'll understand how to connect with them and foster feelings of trust so your relationship is rock solid. Your therapist will start the session without your child because they must connect with you first. They will listen to the various concerns that you have so they can gain some insight into what your child is struggling with and better understand the dynamics of your family.

The next thing is that you must discuss the objectives and goals you are interested in with your therapist. You can't just start without any clear goal in mind. You need to be able to assess how effective the sessions are for your child, and that means figuring out the objectives that you would like to accomplish with your child right from the start. The various goals that you may be concerned with include helping your child become more self-reliant, more confident, better able to accept themselves, better at solving problems and taking responsibility, and so on. Whatever your goals are, they must be measurable, concrete, and observable.

The next thing to expect is for the therapist to explain to you how their behavior in the playroom can help your child accomplish the goals you would like them to. The therapist should clearly explain to you how your child's decision-making process and their ability to control themselves in the playroom will eventually be observed in their attitude outside of the therapy sessions.

Tracking your child's progress with play therapy also means that there must be ongoing consultations. You cannot expect to see changes in just a day or a week of working with your therapist. Every four or five sessions, your therapist checks in with you so that you can both be aware of what progress, if any, your child is making. This way, your therapist will know if they need to make any adjustments in their approach to helping your child achieve the objectives you have set for them. The therapist can also let you know where you may be going wrong and help you adjust.

Challenges to Contend with and How to Overcome Them

You may have to face certain challenges when working with your child to accomplish the goals you have in mind for them. For one thing, you may have to contend with delayed development. You see, some children who take part in play therapy may not develop as quickly as their peers in certain other aspects, such as social skills, language, or regulating emotions. It doesn't necessarily mean that there's something wrong with your child, and you should definitely not make them feel that way. You must understand that the delayed development can make it more challenging for your child to be fully engaged in play therapy. A good therapist would be aware of these delays and would do their best to adjust their methods as needed. Maybe they need to offer simpler instructions for your child to follow. Maybe they need to be more supportive. They may just have to adjust the activities in a way that matches your child. Whether you're a parent or therapist, you must meet the child halfway so they can actually grow and develop.

Another challenge you may deal with is resistance to certain activities. Some children are simply averse to certain activities. It could be because they're afraid, uncomfortable, or just not interested. Your therapist needs to work out why your child is reacting the way they are, and not only that, you must both be respectful of your child's boundaries. If you notice that your child continues to refuse to take part in certain activities, the therapist has to figure out an alternative method or introduce a different activity that's meant to achieve the same results. This way, you develop their trust and make them feel much safer. They will eventually understand that the environment they're in is free of both judgment and criticism. When they realize that, there is a chance they will circle back to the activities they refused to take part in at first.

Sometimes, your child's emotions may be incredibly difficult to manage. Play therapy is all about exploring the different emotions and how they can express them. Even for adults, emotions are challenging. Your child may struggle with trying to figure out what they're feeling, let alone why they're feeling it. On top of that, they may have trouble containing their emotional responses to certain things and explaining how they feel the way they do. Your therapist has to do everything they can to support your child to help them handle the whirlwind of emotions. To do this, your child has to have a safe space to express themselves. You and the therapist must do whatever you can to validate your child's feelings and offer guidance by modeling healthy coping strategies. In the end, they will learn how to communicate what they feel. But you must be patient with them and resist the urge to rush the process.

No one should ever consider all children to be the same, as certain approaches that work for one may not work for another. However, there are certain strategies that tend to work across the board. For one thing, you and the therapist must be flexible and adaptable in your approach. Whatever you do must be tailored to your child's needs and capabilities.

This should go without saying when trying to accomplish things with children, but patience and empathy are absolutely necessary. Children are very sensitive, and they can pick up on when you're irritated or dissatisfied. Having them feel like a burden will only hinder, or even cancel out, any progress you made so far.

Another thing to remember is that the parents and the therapist need to cooperate when handling the issues surrounding the child's life. By doing so, your therapist would be able to see things you may not have noticed before and recommend ways you can be more supportive of your child outside of therapy sessions.

When you engage with your child, you need to be playful at times. The best way to get your little one engaged in the activity is to tailor the experiences to what they prefer and keep their interests in mind. Your therapist will suggest new toys, games, and activities based on your answers to their questions at your first session.

Finally, the therapist you choose must be one who is open to self-reflection and constant supervision. This therapist, ideally, checks in with other therapists to process their experience as they work with your child, to receive new insights, and, where needed, refine their strategy toward helping your child accomplish the goals you set out at the start of your sessions.

Tracking Your Child's Progress

The following is a comprehensive guide to help you track your little one's developmental progress.

1. **Use traditional pen and paper.** You can journal at the end of each day. Write down your observations about your child's behavior. Note any milestones they've hit, challenges they may face, and behaviors they exhibit. Use a calendar to mark the important events or milestones your child hits. A calendar is an excellent tool to visualize their progress over time.

2. **Use digital apps.** You can use spreadsheets like Google Sheets or Excel to track various skills and behaviors your child is exhibiting. Create different categories for these behaviors. Log their observations each week or day using various colors and symbols to show how much progress they're making. Chart their progress with a graph or apps for tracking child development.

3. **Work with behavioral charts.** Whenever your child behaves how you'd like them to, give them a sticker and put it on their chart for them to see. This is a visual way to encourage them to do well each time. Also, develop a behavioral point system. Anytime your child does something well, they get a point. When they've accumulated a set amount of points, you reward them.

4. **Use visual aids.** Take photographs of your child whenever they have accomplished something huge. Photograph their projects, art, and new activities that they're involved in. With time, their development will be evident to you and them. Milestone boxes are also a handy tool. Get a box and put different items such as the first letter they wrote you, their art, and anything significant they have created.

5. **Use standardized testing.** If your child is of school age, test them periodically with a standardized test to see their academic performance.

6. **Get feedback from others.** The people giving you feedback should be trustworthy. Get regular updates from coaches, teachers, tutors, and instructors your child interacts with. This will give you a balanced external perspective and ensure you are not missing something because of how close you are to your child. Feedback can include what other children have to say about your child.

7. **Self-assessment works.** Try using a progress booklet where your child can write or draw whatever they've learned or accomplished each week. This is a great way to encourage them to learn how to self-reflect and become more self-aware. Set a regular time when you and your child can talk about how they feel, what they feel proud of accomplishing, and the obstacles they're facing.

8. **Try structured observation.** While your child plays, observe them. Don't interrupt. Pay attention to any new behaviors they exhibit or new skills they pick up. You may assign them tasks, such as a puzzle, and see how they solve it.

9. **Work with checklists and inventories.** You can create developmental milestone checklists that are age-appropriate. As your child hits each milestone, tick it off. The same applies to behavioral checklists. Pay attention to the skills and behaviors you would like your child to exhibit more, and note when and how they act as you'd prefer.

10. **Use professional evaluation.** Have a pediatrician regularly check up on your child to ensure their physical health is as it should be. Work with counselors or therapists regularly to see how your child is progressing.

These are ways to track your child's progress as you work with them. Remember, you should never compare your child to another. Be as objective as possible regardless of how emotionally involved you are. Whenever there's progress, no matter how little, celebrate it.

If you notice a method of tracking your child's progress isn't working for you, it's okay to change it. You can always tweak these methods to create something that works for you and your baby. The goal of tracking their progress is not to pressure them and make them feel like they're not good enough. You're tracking them to see how you can support their development. So don't rush your child into becoming a runner when they're still learning to crawl.

Conclusion

Of all the jobs that exist to date, parenting continues to be one that is riddled with challenges, twists and turns, and emotional highs and lows. There are so many things to be concerned about regarding how your child grows and develops. You only get a chance to be a parent with any particular child once, and the last thing you want to do is mess it up. So, naturally, you will be nervous and have some trepidation regarding this topic. Today, many values, milestones, and benchmarks indicate certain expectations, which can be a little too overwhelming. You may find yourself giving into the temptation to compare where your child is in life versus other children. Remember, your child is far different from any other, so it would be unreasonable to ask them to develop at the same pace as other children and unfair to make comparisons. As their primary caregiver, you must maintain a positive disposition and remain patient as your child develops into a full-fledged human being. This is not a sprint. It is a marathon, and you must act accordingly.

Play therapy is an excellent way for your child to explore, learn, and grow. With it, you will see their innate identity and that they have the potential to develop into a wonderful person. By using play therapy, your child will be able to express themselves and communicate with others as naturally as possible. In the process of playing, they will become more aware of who they are and learn all about their feelings and how they can handle them. They will be at peace with their choices and understand the processes that led them to be who they are. As their caregiver, you play a crucial role in offering your child support as they continue to progress through life.

One of the major benefits of play therapy is teaching your child to become autonomous, both in and out of the sessions. Your child can be the one in charge of their therapy and should be. There's no room for you to force your opinions on them. The only thing you have a say in is the objective that you would like them to accomplish. How the child accomplishes this in a play therapy session is entirely up to them. You must learn to trust that your child has the innate ability to figure out their development journey at their own pace and in their own way. They have their own unique rhythm, and they will accomplish the goals you've set only when it's time.

You'll have to make peace with the challenges you'll face and do your best to handle them head-on. It's all a natural part of growing up. You just need to be as understanding and supportive as possible and recall that your child's progress is not something that you can rush through. They are not in competition with anyone. It is a personal journey for them, and you must be patient as they discover themselves and develop as a result.

Your job as the primary caregiver or parent is to ensure that they are in a nurturing and supportive environment. You want to make sure they have room to communicate freely with you, that you actively pay attention to them, and that you validate every one of their emotions. Creating the sort of safe, non-critical environment your child needs makes it easier for them to express their concerns, fears, hopes, and dreams. So, you should encourage them to explore the world around them and the one within. Have them celebrate when they've accomplished something, and gently guide them when they feel a little bit lost. That way, you'll be well on your way to turning an adorable little human into a lovely person full of warmth and love.

Check out another book in the series

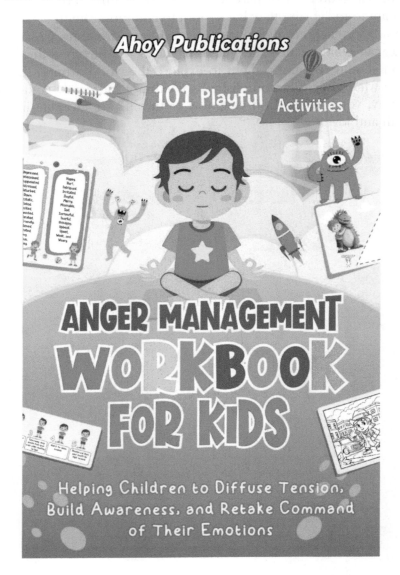

References

American Academy of Family Physicians. (n.d.). How to teach good behavior: Tips for parents. https://www.aafp.org/pubs/afp/issues/2002/1015/p1463.html

As for additional sources on play therapy for toddlers, here are ten books that might be helpful:

Axline, V.M., & Armstrong, H.C. (1969). Play therapy: The inner dynamics of childhood.

Bratton, S.C., Ray, D., Rhine, T., & Jones, L. (2005). The efficacy of play therapy with children: A meta-analytic review of treatment outcomes.

Carmichael, K.D. (2006). Play therapy: An introduction.

Clara. (2022, February 27). 23 Fun Empathy Activities for Kids + (Printable) Kindness Challenge. Very Special Tales. https://veryspecialtales.com/empathy-activities-for-kids-printable-kindness/

Edutopia. (n.d.). Integrating music into social and emotional learning. https://www.edutopia.org/article/integrating-music-social-and-emotional-learning

Foran, L. M. (2009). Listening to music: Helping children regulate their emotions and improve learning in the classroom. Educational Horizons, 88(1), 51-58. https://files.eric.ed.gov/fulltext/EJ868339.pdf

Gil, E., & Drewes, A.A. (2005). Cultural issues in play therapy.

Guerney Jr., L.F., & Guerney, B.G. (1997). Child-centered play therapy.

Healthline (n.d.). Sensory Play: 20 Great Activities for Your Toddler or Preschooler. https://www.healthline.com/health/childrens-health/sensory-play

Homeyer, L.E., & Morrison, M.O. (2008). Play therapy practices, issues, and trends: A sourcebook.

https://www.facebook.com/parents. (2022). The Secret Language of Toddlers: What Their Behaviors Mean. Parents. https://www.parents.com/toddlers-preschoolers/development/behavioral/what-toddler-behavior-means/

https://www.verywellmind.com/play-therapy-definition-types-techniques-5194915

https://www.verywellmind.com/child-development-theories-2795068

Kaduson, H.G., & Schaefer, C.E. (2006). 101 favorite play therapy techniques.

Landreth, G.L., & Bratton, S.C. (1999). Child-centered play therapy.

O'Connor, K.J., & Schaefer, C.E. (1994). Handbook of play therapy.

PositivePsychology.com. (n.d.). 16 activities to stimulate emotional development in children. https://positivepsychology.com/emotional-development-activities/

Rasmussen University (n.d.). 25 Sensational Sensory Activities for Toddlers - Rasmussen University. https://www.rasmussen.edu/degrees/education/blog/sensory-activities-for-toddlers/

Schaefer, C.E., & O'Connor, K.J. (1983). Handbook of Play Therapy

Made in the USA
Monee, IL
22 November 2024

70900620R00044